Marj Pettinger

Straight From The Heart - A Healing Journey

Marj Pettinger

Straight From The Heart - A Healing Journey

Rewriting The Stories of Our Lives with God's Grace, Heuristic Research and Self-Search Inquiry

LAP LAMBERT Academic Publishing

Impressum/Imprint (nur für Deutschland/ only for Germany)
Bibliografische Information der Deutschen Nationalbibliothek: Die Deutsche Nationalbibliothek
verzeichnet diese Publikation in der Deutschen Nationalbibliografie; detaillierte bibliografische
Daten sind im Internet über http://dnb.d-nb.de abrufbar.
Alle in diesem Buch genannten Marken und Produktnamen unterliegen warenzeichen-, marken-
oder patentrechtlichem Schutz bzw. sind Warenzeichen oder eingetragene Warenzeichen der
jeweiligen Inhaber. Die Wiedergabe von Marken, Produktnamen, Gebrauchsnamen,
Handelsnamen, Warenbezeichnungen u.s.w. in diesem Werk berechtigt auch ohne besondere
Kennzeichnung nicht zu der Annahme, dass solche Namen im Sinne der Warenzeichen- und
Markenschutzgesetzgebung als frei zu betrachten wären und daher von jedermann benutzt
werden dürften.

Coverbild: www.ingimage.com

Verlag: LAP LAMBERT Academic Publishing AG & Co. KG
Dudweiler Landstr. 99, 66123 Saarbrücken, Deutschland
Telefon +49 681 3720-310, Telefax +49 681 3720-3109
Email: info@lap-publishing.com

Herstellung in Deutschland:
Schaltungsdienst Lange o.H.G., Berlin
Books on Demand GmbH, Norderstedt
Reha GmbH, Saarbrücken
Amazon Distribution GmbH, Leipzig
ISBN: 978-3-8383-7144-3

Imprint (only for USA, GB)
Bibliographic information published by the Deutsche Nationalbibliothek: The Deutsche
Nationalbibliothek lists this publication in the Deutsche Nationalbibliografie; detailed
bibliographic data are available in the Internet at http://dnb.d-nb.de.
Any brand names and product names mentioned in this book are subject to trademark, brand
or patent protection and are trademarks or registered trademarks of their respective holders.
The use of brand names, product names, common names, trade names, product descriptions
etc. even without a particular marking in this works is in no way to be construed to mean that
such names may be regarded as unrestricted in respect of trademark and brand protection
legislation and could thus be used by anyone.

Cover image: www.ingimage.com

Publisher: LAP LAMBERT Academic Publishing AG & Co. KG
Dudweiler Landstr. 99, 66123 Saarbrücken, Germany
Phone +49 681 3720-310, Fax +49 681 3720-3109
Email: info@lap-publishing.com

Printed in the U.S.A.
Printed in the U.K. by (see last page)
ISBN: 978-3-8383-7144-3

DEDICATION

This Project/Dissertation is dedicated to the Glory of God, the memory of Dr. Richard Laplante with gratitude, to all those needing a word of encouragement in discovering and telling your story, and to all those who minister to the sick and hurting people in our world today.

ACKOWLEDGEMENTS

There are many people to whom I owe a debt of gratitude, people who have walked with me at various stages of completion of my entire doctoral studies process.

Thank you to Dr. Richard Laplante without whose support and encouragement I would not/could not have begun nor completed this work. Even in death, you have been my encouragement.

Thank you to each one who served on my doctoral studies committee. Thank you to Dr. Fran Hare (Liaison), Dr. Leslie Gardner, Virginia Lynn-White and Dr. Geoffrey Wilfong Pritchard. I truly appreciate the insights, the wisdom, the encouragement and the time you all gave so freely. Thank you to former committee members, Dr. Jean Waters and Dr. Marilyn Hundleby and to my friend Michele Raynor, who not only served, for a time, as part of my committee, but also supervised both my major project and my major research.

Thank you to Dr. Rebecca Davis Mathias, who became both my ethical consultant and editor. It was indeed a pleasure to have you journey with me.

Thank you to Doug Thompson, Dr.Yoko Tarumi, Dr. Carol Vogler, Doug Allen, Sandy Smith, Glen Huser, Shirley Serviss, Dawn Rounceville and Ruth Hampton for reading or critiquing various aspects of my work. Although some of that work did not, ultimately find its way into the final dissertation, it was good preparation and your help was much appreciated.

Thank you to Penny and Stan Spence, Dorothy Swan and Maureen Conrad who were all major players in differing ways. Thank you to my colleagues at both St. Stephen's and at Caritas for their support. Thank you to my sisters for the many hours of discussion and challenge. And last but certainly not least a huge thank you to my husband Glen for his

constant support and encouragement. Thank you to each one of you.

TABLE OF CONTENTS

CHAPTER ONE

INTRODUCTION

The Journey Begins

When the night has been too lonely, and the road has been too long...
Just remember in the winter far beneath the bitter snows,
Lies the seed that with the sun's love, in the spring
Becomes the rose (Music and Lyrics by Amanda McBroom, *The Rose 1979).*

There have been times in my journey when it seems as though the night has been too
lonely and the road too long. I invite you to travel with me to yesterday, pause in today and
finally glimpse into tomorrow. I can only appreciate the richness of my journey by looking it
full in the face with all the difficulties and joys. When my experiences are, to paraphrase
Amanda McBroom's words exposed to the sun's rays through telling the stories, opportunity
for growth and healing can blossom and my life is fuller for the experience.

It is the goal of this dissertation to find meaning through story in the experience of
inner healing. The predominant question is "What is the experience of healing as revealed
through story?"

In this introductory chapter I will give an overview of the entire dissertation. The
research is a heuristic self-search inquiry and so I will firstly introduce myself and tell you
just enough of my story to entice you to read on. I will outline my methodology, look at the
concepts of healing and what that means to me, and then discuss briefly the ethical concerns
that arose for me, and the prominent theological themes. I have relied heavily throughout
this dissertation on scripture and have consulted the works of authors such as Louise

DeSalvo, Carl Rodgers, Deena Metzger, Richard Stone, Neville Kirkwood and numerous others.

Throughout this dissertation I have followed the *MLA Handbook for Writers of Research Papers* style of writing. Scripture references are taken from the *New International Version* of the Bible unless otherwise noted.

This dissertation is a *heuristic self-search inquiry.* It is not merely a look at the facts that make up my life, but rather is an in-depth look at who I really am, where I have been and where I hope to go. My "living human document", a phrase coined by Anton Boisen, (qtd. in Asquith 2) reveals the many facets of my world and the many faces of myself which merge into the fabric of who I am.

So, Who Am I Really?

I am the carefree child and the abused frightened child, the defensive rebellious teenager and the poor offspring of an alcoholic father. I am the determined student and I am never quite good enough. I am the young wife and mother and the grieving widow. I am the poet, the storyteller and the listener. I was an early feminist. I am a wife, a mother, a grandmother and a great-grandmother. I am, ultimately a follower of Jesus as I entered the ministry to make a difference and stand for those who cannot stand for themselves. I am all of these and much more.

All stories have a beginning and I begin mine with my name. My given name was Marjorie. Many years ago my grade seven teacher shortened my name to Marj. I realise that if I had had any input, which I didn't, my name would have become Jorie. Jorie sounds gentler while Marj has a harsh ring in my ears and hardly seems to fit the pre-teen little girl I was at the time. Today I know I am both Marj and Jorie. Jorie is my gentler self while Marj is the more prominent, stronger version; perhaps even representing the professional me who is able to deal with whatever is offered in the harsh realities of life. Jorie represents my feeling side; that aspect of me that moves from head to heart and allows the artistic me to emerge. And yet both aspects of my name fit and each is a reflection of the all of who I am.

A few years back my youngest sister gave me a parchment with Marjorie on it followed by a definition of the name and a scripture verse.

Marjorie
(A Precious Pearl)

I will praise thee, for I am fearfully
and wonderfully made…How precious
also are thy thoughts unto me, O God (Psalm 139:14,17a).

Perhaps for the first time in my life I truly appreciated my name and connected it with who I am in God's eyes. It became more than simply a name my parents had chosen for me; one that I shared with my dad's older sister. My name was changed without any consultation with me. I didn't appear to have any say in the matter. That fact is significant because as a child, I often felt at the mercy of those in power over me. Life's experience created the MARJ of who I am. I recognize the name God gave me. It is mine. God has called me, Marjorie, by name. "Fear not, for I have redeemed you; I have summoned you by name; you are mine" (Isaiah 43:1b). There is resurrection power that has both Biblical roots and feminist roots in naming something or in recognizing and claiming my name as part of my identity. The sound of my name is sweeter as I envision myself through God's eyes and encounter again the Risen Lord. I can wear Marjorie with pride and accept that both Marj and Jorie combine to proclaim my God given identity.

Jesus attached importance to Simon Peter's name as he changed it from Simon to Peter.

> These are the twelve he appointed: Simon (to whom He gave the name
> Peter)…" (Mark 3:16) "The use of the Semitic name Cephas in the post-
> Resurrection appearance to Peter bears witness to the time when the name-
> changing took place, suggesting that it was as the risen Lord showed Himself
> to 'Simon' (cf. Luke. 24:34: "The Lord has risen indeed, and has appeared to
> Simon") that Simon became Cephas (or Peter, as the name rendered into
> Greek) (Bromiley177).

The connection between Peter's name change and his character change seems evident as we read in Matthew's gospel the importance of his confession and the change from Simon to Peter meaning rock. Jesus said, "I also say to you that you are Peter, and upon this rock I will build my church; and the gates of Hades will not overpower it" (Matthew 16:18). Jesus recognized both the strengths and weaknesses in his friend Simon Peter in naming him the rock, which was to be the foundation of the Christian Church. But Peter was human. He wavered at times in his beliefs and even denied that which he knew to be true. In Matthew 26 we see that Peter denied Jesus, not once, but three times and still was used by God in ministry. We all have fallen short of the glory of God –not only Marj. There is freedom in knowing that I, like Peter, can waver, question and even deny and yet come back to that place of grace, mercy and pardon. So, I don't need to be perfect. I can be myself, with all my strengths and weaknesses, in all my humanity, and do that which God has called me to do.

But I am much more than a name. I am the voice of one crying in the wilderness (John 1:23) for I did not always have a voice. As a child I was to be seen and not heard. My voice was silenced in an environment of alcoholism, poverty and abuse.

Tamar's story from 2 Samuel is a reminder that female abuse has spanned the centuries. Women, then as now, at the worst of times, are seen as objects for men's pleasure.

I, like Tamar, was abused by one of my brothers. Both of us were silenced into keeping the secret. A code of silence, along with justifying the abuse, seems to exist in dysfunctional families in which children are coerced into keeping the family secrets within the walls of the household.

Although I am more that merely my name or my voice, both of these aspects have carried considerable weight in the formation of who I have become. I am a name, a voice and an individual who is created in God's image. My formative years were in rural Saskatchewan where I was an unwilling farm girl in a family of twelve. Today I would claim to be a survivor although I now know that for many years I saw myself as a victim, a victim of life itself. I survived the poverty of growing up in a poor farm family with an alcoholic father and a mother who was an enabler in every sense of the word. I was a victim of incest and abuse but perhaps the greatest victimization was my own perception of how things should have been. I let myself be victimized by my own expectations, poor self-image, and a sense of feeling sorry for myself. My grandfather used to say I had a chip on my shoulder and perhaps I did. I had to conquer the demons that played in my mind as the old tapes, such as stupid, poor Whitfield brat, never amount to anything, not good enough, played over and over again like broken records on a gramophone.

I'm not even sure I like the term "survivor" and perhaps would prefer to say I am a conqueror. Scripture tells us we are more than conquerors. "No, in all these things we are more than conquerors through him who loved us" (Romans 8:37). These words give me the assurance that I so desperately need as I journey towards wholeness and ultimately towards accepting myself and knowing, as Carl Rogers so eloquently states, "What I am is good enough if only I would be it openly" (http://www.spiritsong.com/quotes/).

My story is the complex integration of Marj and Jorie combined to form the totality of the person-hood of Marjorie, my whole self. I have lived for over sixty years. I have travelled a great deal and seen many things. I have loved much. Life has, for the most part, been good. My story is one that encompasses all aspects of a life lived to the fullest; a life that witnesses to a faith in a loving God who is there when cruel realities overshadow dreams and visions. As a child I sought refuge in the belief that a loving God somehow protected and cared for me as I heard the Biblical stories and knew in my innermost being that they were real. That was my lifeline, my hope and my strength.

Stories are, and have always been, an essential ingredient in my life. At the tender age of four I developed a thirst for knowledge. I listened to the Bible Stories through the "Back to the Bible" broadcast on a local radio station and my love affair with stories began. I developed a deep appreciation for the written word in my elementary school years. Like a starving, abandoned cub, I devoured everything I could lay my hands on, mostly biographies and real life stories of people who lived lives that were much more exciting than mine. I grew up on the stories of others but learned early that I, too, had a story to tell. I realized, even as a child, that there was true value in both telling and writing my experiences.

Boisen, credited with being the founder of the Clinical Pastoral Education (CPE) model of chaplaincy training, coined the term "living human document" (Asquith 2). This training introduced me to the concept of each of us being the product of our stories. Writing has allowed me to take that living human document, put words to the traumatic experiences of my life and in self-dialogue become aware of both the healing and the learning. In retrospect I recognize that much of my inner healing has been precipitated not only through the writing of my own story but also through the telling, the reading, the sharing and the listening.

My passion for story and writing continues today. My inner search inquiry has challenged me to seek what Clark Moustakas refers to as an "unwavering and steady inward gaze and inner freedom to explore and accept what is" (*Heuristic Research* 13). It is difficult for me to be vulnerable and to reveal those memories that I have kept silently hidden behind closed doors for so long. I have to confront my fears and be willing to accept whatever unfolds, as I look inward. "The fear of self discovery is a strong component in avoiding loneliness & solitude. Once this courageous step is taken, however, there is no turning back" (Moustakas, *Touch of Loneliness* 22). Unlike Moustakas, I find the urge to turn back at times overwhelming. It is an urge I struggle to resist. Sandy Sela-Smith, in her methodology, notes that "resistance" (84) is the primary reason people cannot stay in the feeling self that is required in heuristic self-search inquiry. Revisiting traumatic events in my life takes both courage and inner strength before those moments can surface in which my own inner healing is possible. My inner healing and transformation comes with a shift of attitude or a change in a relationship as I overcome and move through the resistance. I cannot do it alone but go forward with faith and trust in the presence of God. Sometimes I feel God's presence while other times I hear God's voice. Even in those times when I want to ask, "God, where are you?" I put my faith and trust in the assurance that God will never leave me nor forsake me (Hebrews 13:5). That trust is reflected in a deep sense of inner peace. It is the peace that passes all understanding as spoken of in Philippians 4:7.

The Dissertation Research Process

The research process explored in detail in "Chapter Two – Methodology," combined Moustakas' heuristic research, Sela-Smith's self-search inquiry and an ethical component. The process involved an exploration of self, which stemmed from opening myself to learning and perhaps more importantly, to feeling, and allowing myself to flow in the feeling and let it inform me. This involved a new and challenging way of learning for me. My growing need to discover the response to my research question from an internal perspective became the driving force for me to explore exactly what healing through story was for me and allow the process to lead wherever it might.

In each lifetime there are those defining moments of time that stand out for us. Earlier in the doctoral studies program we were asked to complete a time line of milestones in our lives. These events consisted of experiences that shaped us and perhaps set the direction for our lives. It was now time to revisit those defining moments such as abuse, leaving home, marriage, deaths and births, to determine which particular experiences contributed towards my inner healing or perhaps merely cried out to be told through story and possibly invite healing in the telling.

A Personal Introduction to Heuristics

I was introduced to heuristics early in my Clinical Pastoral Education training and then again as I entered the doctoral studies program and enrolled in the Qualitative Research course. For my Major Applied Research project, which is a prerequisite to the Project Dissertation proposal formation in the Doctor of Ministry program, I developed my research question, which was, "In the artist's viewpoint, what experience of God and Spiritual healing, if any, is revealed by patients through their artistic expression?" The qualitative research methodology was phenomenological. In that context the assumption I made was that there is indeed a connection between theology, art and healing. Both heuristic and narrative methodologies fall within the scope of phenomenological research and I used both of those in my research. Moustakas' methodology, that encourages the use of personal investigation or observation, became the foundation for my research engaging co-researchers from the "artists on the ward" program at the University Hospital. The research was completed and received committee approval in 2002.

Earlier in the Doctor of Ministry program, my Major Supervised Project guided me to discover new insights about myself as I undertook the task of writing, compiling and publishing a book of poetry. I had written poetry as a child but had never before shared it with anyone or explored, in any depth, the significance of poetry or writing in healing. I enrolled in classes and attended a poetry convention in Washington, D.C., after having poetry published by the Famous Poet's Society. I received the "Editor's Choice" award of distinction for one of my poems. That convention was a launching pad for my creative juices and I began to write more extensively. Each step of the Doctoral Studies led to the next step and became part of my inner healing journey.

It seemed natural then, after discussion with my committee, to follow through and utilize heuristic research as the methodology of choice for my dissertation. Chapter two outlines in detail how I combined both Moustakas' and Sela-Smith's methodologies to establish the foundation for my research for this dissertation.

Ethical Considerations

Throughout this process of self-search inquiry I came face-to-face with some rather intense ethical questions. I needed to tell my stories. But these stories are not mine alone. The stories, of necessity, include family members and others who may be impacted as the stories unfold. In my inner healing journey it has been necessary at times to "air our dirty laundry in public." The family secrets that were kept closely guarded behind closed doors came to light for all to see. Ethical concerns arose as I thought about the possible damage, or repercussions, that my stories may have on others. I know that truth does not damage, rather it rectifies or heals the damage. There is freedom in truth and with freedom comes healing. "The truth shall set you free" (John 8:30). My stories have helped me to become the person I have become. I am bigger than any one part of my experience, for I am the sum total of all those experiences. I realize that my remembrances of my childhood and my life are specific to me. Even my siblings who lived through the same experiences will have their own memories of those events. It is not my intent to create discord in the lives of persons who might see themselves in my stories. It is rather the intent that my stories might encourage others to tell their stories and journey towards wholeness through their own inner healing.

The Health Research Ethics Board (HREB) advised me that I did not need to submit my research to them since it was an internal research that did not involve outside co-researchers or subjects. However, as I wrote my own healing journey, I still had questions about the detrimental affects telling my stories could have on family members, both present and future. Dr. Rebecca Davis Mathias, Assistant Professor at St. Joseph's College, University of Alberta, who also serves as an ethicist with Caritas Health Group and St. Joseph's Auxiliary Hospital, agreed to journey with me as I struggled with ethical issues.

With guidance and prayerful discernment I have been able to move forward trusting that the written revealed word of my stories will be healing and freeing for myself and others.

Healing from the Inside Out

Step into my world, the world of Marjorie, Marj and Jorie as I explore my own inner-healing journey. It is an exploration of the healing in my life and the importance of story in the recognition of that healing. I deal with healing, not in the physical sense, but in the emotional and spiritual sense, although I recognize that body, soul and spirit are not mutually exclusive.

A primary assumption is that the sharing of experience through story opens the door to healing. It is not the story itself that heals but rather that the story serves as an agent for healing. I make this conclusion based on having experienced this to be true in my own life. The assumption is recognized in the field of chaplaincy and is beginning to gain more credibility within the overall medical community. I have facilitated grief groups and other adult self-help groups in which telling one's story is a vital ingredient and fosters healing.

Story is important to me. I am a storyteller. I am a story listener. Story is who I am and what I do. As researcher I returned to my childhood memories of abuse, ridicule and lack of self-esteem.

There was an inner struggle as I went about the task of reflection and inner search. I was forced to question my own perception, my own truth, on what I remembered and those memories that have shaped my life. I was not beaten; I was not starved, at least not in any physical sense, but there are other kinds of abuse and pain. My pain was very real. As I let my mind be totally absorbed, I broke out in a cold sweat and wondered if it was simply menopausal, but no I'm past that, and then I recognized my fear of revisiting memories and my denial of the reality of my experiences. I didn't want to go there and I wondered about many things. I realized the necessity of forgiving my dad before I could publish my book of poetry. I wondered about that and questioned what it was I had to forgive him for and what healing still needed to take place. All of this was part of the painful process.

Healing Defined

Holistic healing is the mantle upon which healing is hung throughout this dissertation. Perhaps Tomas D. Maddix and Ian C. Soles come closest to what I mean by their words,

> When we speak of healing, we mean a sense of well-being and wholeness. We do not mean cure of illness or disease, but a sense of acceptance. Healing brings the fragments of our life together as a whole, and frees our spirits to be about their business (11).

To achieve that sense of acceptance referred to by Maddix and Soles takes time and effort. Today's medical community, of which I am a part, is giving more credence to holistic healing as we work together as multi-disciplinary teams to achieve a measure of wholeness or health that recognizes the entire person as body, soul and spirit.

Thomas R. Egnew, in his qualitative inquiry, interviewed prominent physicians including Eric J. Cassell, Carl A. Hammerschlag, Elizabeth Kubler Ross and Bernard S. Siegel, whose works have involved the study of healing. The objective of Egnew's study was "to determine a definition of healing that operationalizes its mechanisms and thereby identifies those repeatable actions that reliably assist physicians to promote holistic healing" (1). Within the context of this inquiry Cassell said, "To be whole again is to be in

relationship to yourself...to your body, to the culture and significant others" (4).
Hammerschlag said ... it is possible to be in health and to be healed without being cured" (4),
while Siegel noted that healing is "a reinterpretation, in a sense, of life" (4). In summary,
Egnew concluded his abstract by stating that, "Healing may be operationally defined as the
personal experience of the transcendence of suffering" (1). There is recognition that health is
more than merely a physical state of well-being and that healing is more than a cure.

In Biblical times, healing referred to the well-being of the entire person and then with
medical advances the focus shifted to more concentration on physical healing.

> The basic element in the concept of the health of human beings in the Old
> Testament and in the Bible as a whole is that of relationship ... for which the
> keyword is righteousness. In other words, well-being consists of right
> relationships (John Wilkinson 19).

Wilkinson's thoughts echo those of Cassell. Both concur with the concept that we, as
human beings are much more than our physical beings. We are spirit, soul and body—each
aspect equally important and connected through right relationship. Our well-being then,
depends not only on ourselves but also on those with whom we are in relationship. These
people are part of the fabric of our lives. They are part of our stories.

Telling our stories empowers us to open to the fullness of life. My stories invite me
to a deeper self-understanding as I remember, record, share and reframe my experiences
recognizing that as Metzger says,

> Every life is a story. Telling the story and seeing our life as story are part of
> the creative process ... Sometimes the simple willingness to explore story
> asserts the reality of the individual, and then the creative process of finding
> and telling the story becomes part of the way that we construct a life (49).

Stories can be healing as we become whole through the telling. In the process of writing, of discovering our story, we restore those parts of ourselves that have been scattered, hidden, suppressed, denied, distorted or forbidden, and we come to understand that stories heal. The title of Metzger's book, *Writing for Your Life,* brings a sense of urgency. The image for me is one in which the writer is frantically writing the stories and it is a matter of life or death. The writing will sustain life while silence around unspoken secrets speaks of death of my childhood and my spirit.

I am energized as I write and realize that I am creating my story anew. I am taking past experiences, revisiting and reframing them and as I do so I am recreating my past. "'Creativity' says psychoanalyst Dr. John Rickmann, cited in Wolin and Wolin, 'is building a new world on the ruins of the old. The promise of renewal pushes many resilient survivors in creative directions'" (177). Both Metzger and Wolin and Wolin speak of creating something new out of the old. The conceptual image for me is that of resurrection as new life springs forth from the old and a movement towards healing begins. Revisiting my family farm as recorded in Chapter Three, "Through The Eyes of a Child," was a process of building a new world from the ruins of my old world. I reframed the experience and rewrote it as memories filled in the gaps to round out the story and create my new reality.

DeSalvo tells us that it is not merely a matter of writing but rather,

> Writing that describes traumatic or distressing events in detail *and* how we felt about these events then and feel about them now is the only kind of writing about trauma that clinically has been associated with improved health … Both thinking and feeling are involved. Linking them is crucial (25).

DeSalvo has just described an essential component of the heuristic process

that I am undertaking for this dissertation. It was necessary for me to allow the
integration of the "I who feels" (Sela-Smith 57), as I journeyed back, almost reliving
the experiences, and the "I who observes" as I reflected on what it was like to both
revisit and write the stories of my inner healing journey.

Richard Stone claims that through the act of telling the story we are changed in how
we see events and how we feel in relation to those events. Telling the story takes the "stuff
of suffering and transforms it into one of the most elemental and important materials of
human existence - meaning" (47). This concept is similar to that which Wolin and Wolin
talk about as "building a new world out of the ruins of the old" (177), as both of them along
with Metzger, refer to rebuilding or re-constructing our stories. As I revisited my
experiences and retold my stories, the memories became more than the pain of past hurts as
other memories claimed space and the greater reality of all the experience came into being
and I changed my perception of the story.

Telling the story allows me to move from being the victim of circumstances beyond
my control. Listening is the other side of the equation and is equally as important as the
telling. "Real listening is the creation of a sacred space in which another's words are
contained and transformed into hallowed speech. Like remembering, this form of listening is
also intentional" (Stone 54). I had to listen to the memories and as I read and reread my own
stories, I had to listen as though hearing them for the first time.

This dissertation is recognition of a personal healing journey. "Healing and
integration do not occur overnight. Instead, the process of healing and integrating our mind,
body and soul is a journey - not a destination" (Maddix and Soles 119). Maddix and Soles, in
describing what they refer to as a journey to wholeness and without using the terminology

holistic healing describe the context in which I use the term healing throughout this dissertation. In chapter 11 of their book they speak to "Integrating the fragments of our lives" (119). Soles states that in his experience "I have noted that the deep, lasting peace that comes from living a congruent, integrated life comes only with reconciling all parts of ourselves" (123), and he then goes on to say, "The longing for wholeness shapes our lives whether or not we are conscious of it" (129). That longing for wholeness is my ultimate goal and this dissertation is part of that journey.

Each of the authors referenced above recognizes that holistic healing relates to the entire person and that the perceptions we hold of ourselves, and the world around us, play significant roles in our overall wholeness.

Theological Reflection

As I moved to deeper levels of theological exploration I was challenged to examine my own beliefs. My background is very eclectic with roots in The Roman Catholic, Anglican, United, and ultimately Pentecostal churches. The ability to interact ecumenically is part of the blessing of such a rich heritage. But within that milieu there are challenges and theological reflection allows me to explore and to seek further understanding. Attending a liberal theological college to complete this doctorate was part of the challenge to re-examine my belief system. My Bachelor of Theology was completed at The Pentecostal Assemblies Theological College and my Masters was completed at the Baptist Seminary. This gave me a firm foundation in conservative theology and the courage to look towards St. Stephen's liberal theological college for my doctorate. In hindsight, this experience, and the works of others, have sharpened my growing edges and invited transformation in my inner healing journey. As I sought to determine which theological themes were predominant in my life and my ministry I read the works of Paul Jones, Patricia O'Connell Killen and John DeBeer, Earle Cairns, Hendrikus Berkhof, and Mathew Fox. All of this, along with my theological education and chaplaincy training has deepened my theology. I have been challenged to dialogue with other perspectives and as a chaplain, to interact and minister to those of different faiths. "As iron sharpens iron, so one person sharpens another" (Proverbs 27:17).

Theological reflection has strengthened my faith and given me courage to give voice to that which I hold to be true. Dr. Richard Laplante, who was the coordinator of the Doctor of Ministry program at the time I entered St. Stephen's College, expressed his hope for me in these words, "It would be my hope for you that St. Stephen's would make you a better Pentecostal, not that they would make you a liberal theologian." These words took on a deep significance for me. I believe that hope has come to fruition with the result that I am more comfortable and at ease with who I am in Christ Jesus. In the process I have gained a better understanding of my more liberal colleagues. It is acceptable for us to disagree. The importance is in the relationship and the resulting conversation.

Story Theology stands out as the encompassing thread, which ties together *relational theology, transformational theology, experiential or lived theology, and a theology of forgiveness,* as the foundations for my life, my ministry and this dissertation. We are our stories and each of these themes is part of the story of my life revealed in the pages of this dissertation. The scriptures are full of stories of the lives of people in Biblical times, which relate to my own life.

Life, in its entirety, for me revolves around the many relationships in my life and thus *Relational Theology,* "A term that embraces a variety of expressions of emphasis on

interpersonal relationships as central to one's theological outlook" (Donald K. McKim 235),
is a natural part of the formation of my life and ministry. Reflecting theologically allows me
to bring my life, with all those relationships, into conversation with my Christian heritage.
"It is not good for man to be alone ..." (Genesis 2:18), indicates that it was God's desire for
human relationships. And so we are put into families, not of our own choosing. Some of
those families prove to be relatively healthy while others are more dysfunctional. The
scriptures reveal numerous relationships, some healthy, some unhealthy, which remind me
that while dysfunction as a word might be relatively new, as a concept it is as old as time.

Both my Roman Catholic maternal grandmother and an evangelical cousin were
instrumental in my early faith development. My grandmother's prayer life and my cousin's
commitment to his beliefs were strong influences in my childhood. I witnessed my
grandmother on her knees in prayer morning and night as I spent time at her home during
summer vacations. My cousin, on the other hand, would share the bible stories with us when
he came to visit us. He was ten years my senior and I always looked forward to the times
when he visited our farm. Both these relationships impacted the formation of my belief
system.

Transformational Theology continues to be part of my journey. Each new experience
brings with it opportunity for new growth and holds possibility for transformation. Stories
throughout scripture reveal transformation in the lives of our Biblical ancestors in which the
stories read our lives and we can dialogue with the scripture as we see similarities within our
own stories. The story of Joseph, in Genesis 37, and the story of Tamar in 2 Samuel 13, are
two such examples in which I can bring my own life story into my Christian heritage and
relate to the people of Biblical times.

As we read the story of Joseph and his family we see that Joseph's brothers were jealous of his gifts and his relationship with his father, Jacob. They mocked him, abused him, mistreated him and sold him into slavery and yet ultimately we witness transformation in many lives. We see forgiveness and a change in attitude. I relate to the story of Joseph, perhaps with wistfulness in desiring to have experienced a relationship of favor with my father such as that of Joseph and Jacob. Joseph was wronged and forgave those who wronged him. It is my desire to live my life reflecting a theology of forgiveness as I pray, "forgive me my trespasses as I forgive those who trespass against me" (Matthew 6:12).

Aspects of Tamar's story, read my life, as both of us suffered abuse at the hands of one of our brothers. Abuse always brings transformation, not of our own choosing, but rather that, which is forced upon us. Ultimately we choose how we allow circumstances to effect our attitudes towards life and we act according to those choices. Transformation does not always happen instantaneously and so, I continue to be encouraged as I reflect on difficult or trying times in my own life and know that positive transformation can happen.

Experiential, or Lived Theology is sometimes referred to as a theology of experience in which "theology is based on one's own experience rather than on an external authority" (*Westminster Dictionary of Theological Terms* 99). Mary Magdalene's faith was definitely shaped by her experience. In (John 20:10) Mary encountered Jesus firsthand and became the first evangelist as she left the tomb and went announcing to the disciples that she had seen the Lord. The theology of noted theologians such as Martin Luther and John Wesley was influenced by their personal experience.

Similarly, my experiences through spiritual encounters with the Holy Spirit and the person of Jesus have shaped my theology. The impact of the *Back to the Bible* radio broadcasts during my childhood years is not something that can be readily explained. I experienced Christ and the love of God through those radio waves and my life was impacted.

It is my hope that beyond each experience exists the possibility of growth, healing and resurrection. In many ways I have died to the old self I used to be. Life has not been easy and at times I have been overwhelmed and wondered where I could find the strength to carry on. I am encouraged by the words of the Apostle Paul, "I can do everything through him who gives me strength" (Philippians 4:13). As I lived through the indignities of poverty and alcohol abuse, the death of a brother and of a husband, each experience has strengthened me and prepared me to face the future and whatever that might hold for me. As I look back at my experiences and retell my stories, I can see how "… in all things God works for the good of those who love him …" (Romans 8:28).

Forgiveness has played, and continues to play, a significant role in my life and so I attempt to live a *theology of forgiveness.* As Jesus hung on the cross, he said, "Father, forgive them; for they do not know what they are doing" (Luke 23:34). Likewise the thief on the cross was forgiven. "Then, he said, 'Jesus, remember me when you come into your kingdom.' Jesus answered him, 'I tell you the truth, today you will be with me in paradise'" (Luke 23:42-43). These words demonstrate the power of forgiveness. It is a concept that I need to look at constantly in both the extending and the receiving of the same. God's forgiveness of us through Jesus reminds me that if we are truly created in God's image, and I believe that we are, then we need to be both loving and forgiving as we live according to God's will for our lives. I have struggled with the concept of forgiveness, both in forgiving myself and extending that forgiveness to family members. The last poem I wrote for inclusion in my book of poetry was entitled "Forgiveness" (46) and was written specifically for my dad after his death. Although, prior to that, my major project seemed to be completed and ready to go to publication, I found I was unable to take that step to deliver it to the publisher. The strained relationship between my father and me colored much of my growing up years and there was immense need for forgiveness and healing. Much progress has been made; there is still work to do.

These theological themes of story, relationship, transformation, experience and forgiveness are all part of the foundation of my life and my ministry. Chapter five deals extensively with how those themes have shaped my life.

Summary

I have outlined in this chapter how my dissertation will unfold. I began by sharing some of my history in which I explored the importance of my name and how that has shaped my life. Both my passion for story and my resistance to sharing certain aspects of my story are part of this introduction. Next I set out the methodology I used in my research, being a combination of Moustakas' Heuristic Research and Sela-Smith's Heuristic Self-Search inquiry to which I added an ethical component. I explored my concept of healing in conjunction with definitions from other sources. The ethical considerations section highlighted areas of concern that arose for me and outlined how those would be addressed. The theological reflection portion begins to look at some of the theologies that are operative in my life and my ministry. Each of these sub-sections helps to set the stage for my heuristic self-search inquiry and is dealt with extensively in the body of the dissertation.

CHAPTER TWO

METHODOLOGY

In this chapter I will go through the steps of research by outlining and explaining the two research methodologies I have followed in my process of heuristic self-search inquiry. I will then take the reader through my own process as I went through the various stages.

This dissertation is a heuristic *self-search inquiry* (Sela-Smith) in which I have looked at the question of "what is the experience of healing as revealed through story?" I sought to discover what, if any, healing had occurred for me as I revisited traumatic experiences in my life, wrote stories about those experiences and then shared those stories with others.

I used a combination of the methodologies of Moustakas and Sela-Smith, both proponents of heuristics, and added another component in which, because of the specific nature of my self-search inquiry, I invited a Christian moral ethicist to journey with me.

> The root meaning of *heuristic* comes from the Greek word *heuriskein,* meaning to discover or to find. It refers to a process of internal search through which one discovers the nature and meaning of experience and develops methods and procedures for further investigation and analysis (Moustakas 9).

This internal search, referred to by Moustakas, is foundational to the development of the methodologies of both Moustakas and Sela-Smith, which I have used throughout my heuristic self-search inquiry. Although I have utilized Moustakas' phases, concepts, processes and validation of heuristic research extensively, I found that Moustakas relied heavily on co-researchers in his research design, methodology, examples and application (Moustakas 38-124). I preferred to have a more internal focus in keeping with Sela-Smith's interpretation of heuristic self-search inquiry in which she refers to the "I-who feels" (Sela-

Smith 85), being internally focused compared to the "I-who-observes" being externally focused. Co-researchers create that shift in focus away from an internal inquiry or search.

Moustakas developed six phases of heuristic research and while I have utilized these to guide me through the process, I concur with Sela-Smith, who says,

> The researcher must remain internally focused and dwell within the feelings of the tacit dimension, allowing the six phases to unfold naturally by surrendering to the feeling state of the subjective 'I'... Although the phases must be completed, the completion of the phases cannot be the focus ... If a verbal thought is the focus, the process will be mechanistic; only feeling can direct the process through the uncharted territory to global experience of the tacit dimension (Sela-Smith 63).

In her critique of Moustakas' method, Sela-Smith devotes several pages (Sela-Smith 64-68) to a careful restatement of his six phases. I borrowed heavily from Sela-Smith's version, which I summarize below.

The purpose of the first phase of initial engagement is to discover that inner passion that calls one to action in the form of research. This phase leads the researcher to explore and discover, through "an intense interest, a passionate concern" (Sela-Smith 64), the topic and formulate the question through inner search and dialogue. "During this process, the researcher encounters himself or herself in a way that is autobiographical and touches significant relationships within their social context ... This phase is like the attention-getting circumstance pointing to something that cannot yet be seen but has the *smell* of significance that draws one into inquiry" (Sela-Smith 64-65).

Immersion is the phase in which the researcher "lives the question consciously and unconsciously" (Sela-Smith 65). The question becomes all encompassing and absorbs every waking hour, every sleeping hour and even the dreaming hours. "Everything in his or her life becomes crystallized around the question" (Moustakas 28). The researcher becomes intimately involved with the question, lives the question and thus grows in knowledge and understanding. When the question has been properly formed, it appears to absorb every aspect of life and the question is ever present.

Incubation is the process, in "which the researcher retreats from the intense, concentrated, conscious focus on the question and allows the inner tacit dimension to wrestle with new input gained during immersion, reorganizing and re-forming … creating new meaning, new behaviours and new feelings" (Sela-Smith 67). This is a time for stepping back and allowing new discoveries to begin to formulate.

Illumination "occurs naturally when the researcher is receptive to discovering what exists in the tacit knowledge and intuition" (Sela-Smith 67). It is that moment when there is a breakthrough into conscious awareness that may bring to light new interpretations and meanings, or may correct previously distorted understandings.

The purpose of explication is to fully examine what has, "awakened in deep consciousness" (Sela-Smith 68), in order to understand the various layers of meaning. The entire process of explication requires the researcher to pay close attention to his/her "own awareness, feelings, thoughts, beliefs, and judgments as a prelude to the understanding that can happen in conversations and dialogues with others" (Sela-Smith 68). This brings with it the opportunity to understand more fully and to allow "new insight, new understanding, new meaning, and a new worldview" (Sela-Smith 68) to become part of the researcher.

Creative synthesis is the comprehensive expression of the research and according to Moustakas "usually takes the form of a narrative depiction and allows for the outward expression of the components and core themes … but it may be expressed as a poem, story, drawing, painting, or by some other creative form … the creative synthesis can only be achieved through tacit and intuitive powers" (Moustakas 31-32). This "final phase spontaneously occurs to form a creative synthesis ... This synthesis embodies an inclusive expression of the essences of what has been investigated. It tells the 'story' that reveals some new whole that has been identified and experienced as a result of this union of the deep-consciousness and the waking consciousness and between the internal and the external" (Sela-Smith 68).

Validation claims a category unto itself, separate from either the phases of heuristic research or the concepts and processes, but it is nevertheless a vitally important concept. "Validity of the research is established by the process that is pushing itself into the consciousness of the researcher, allowing the process to unfold and then noticing results in expansion of self-awareness, deepening of self-understanding, and of self-transformation that others can experience in the 'story'" (Sela-Smith 79). "Since heuristic inquiry utilizes qualitative methodology in arriving at themes and essences of experience, validity in heuristics is not a quantitative measurement that can be determined by correlations or statistics. The question of validation is one of meaning" (Moustakas 32). Validation is subjective and depends on the validity of the judgment and interpretation of the researcher. Judgment as to the ultimate depiction of the experience and of both the presentation of meanings and the depth of the experience is the responsibility of the researcher (Moustakas 32-34).

Moustakas identifies various concepts and processes present throughout the entire Process:

- Identifying with the focus of inquiry or getting inside the question and becoming one with it

- Self-dialogue or allowing the phenomenon to speak directly to one's own experience and being open to self-discovery and awareness

- Tacit knowing in which we know more than we can tell. We know something without understanding why we know it

- Intuition in which one utilizes an internal capacity to make inferences and arrive at knowledge

- Indwelling refers to the heuristic process of turning inward to seek deeper understanding of the experience

- Focusing is an inner attention, a staying with the process, clearing an inward space to enable one to tap into thoughts and feelings and the essence of what matters

- Internal frame of reference in which everything is filtered through the lens of the person who has had the experience (Moustakas 15-26).

He argues that the three "crucial processes in heuristics (once one understands the values, beliefs, and knowledge inherent in the heuristic paradigm) are: *concentrated gazing* on something that attracts or compels one into a search for meaning; *focus on a topic* or formulation of the question; and *methods* of preparing, collecting, organizing, analyzing, and synthesizing data" (Moustakas 39). These crucial processes are integrated into the process at appropriate stages throughout.

Sela-Smith worked with Moustakas' methodology to develop a heuristic self-search inquiry in which she concludes there are six key components intrinsic to heuristic inquiry:

- The researcher has experienced what is identified as being researched

- The researcher makes reference to some intense or passionate concern that causes the investigator to *reach inward* for tacit awareness and knowledge

- The research indicates surrender to the question has taken place (living, waking, sleeping, and dreaming the question)

- Self-dialogue, not simply a one-way reporting of thoughts or feelings is evidenced. To report a feeling is not the same as dialoguing with the feeling

- The search is a self-search

- There is evidence that transformation has taken place by way of a "story" that contains the transformation and may transform those who "read" it (Sela-Smith 69).

As part of Sela-Smith's heuristic self-search inquiry, she integrated her threefold application of heuristic research into Moustakas' methodology in attempts to further emphasizes the "self" of heuristic research:

- First, there must be recognition of the value of a *heuristic self-search inquiry* and a return to the internal perspective

- Second, there must be an acknowledgement of resistance to feeling in the reconnection with the *I-who-feels*

- Finally, there must be an acceptance of surrender that opens to transformation that can impact the individual, society and all of humankind (Sela-Smith 85).

Moustakas is widely recognized for his development of the heuristic research methodology, while Sela-Smith expanded on his methodology and brings an interesting perspective that proved to fit for the work of my dissertation. Together these methodologies permitted the flexibility I sought in exploring my own experiences. Sela-Smith's methodology supplied a more complete framework for my own inner search in which I as researcher "encounter myself in a way that is autobiographical and touches significant relationships within the social context" (Moustakas 27, Sela-Smith 64).

As Moustakas moved into "Research Design and Methodology" (38), he states "A typical way of gathering material is through interviews that often take the form of dialogues…with one's research participants" (39). I struggled to understand this aspect of

Moustakas' methodology as he introduced the concept of interviewing co-researchers in a methodology in which he claims, "From the beginning, and throughout the investigation, heuristic research involves *self-search, self-dialogue, and self-discovery; the research question and the methodology flow out of inner awareness, meaning, and inspiration"* (11). Moustakas further states that, "The focus in a heuristic quest is on recreation of the lived experience; full and complete depictions of the experience from the frame of reference of the experiencing person" (39). It is not my intention to critique Moustakas' methodology nor to highlight weaknesses therein but simply to say that before embarking totally into Moustakas' phases of heuristic research methodology I was drawn to Sela-Smith's critique of Moustakas. She stressed the importance of *"recognition of the value of a heuristic self-search inquiry* and a return to the internal perspective" (85). Returning to an internal perspective spoke directly to the shift I made in moving from telling the stories of others to telling my own inner healing journey. My focus shifted from external to internal and my desire to discover and understand the complexities of my life became apparent.

I had to deal with the *"acknowledgement of resistance to feeling in the reconnection with the I-who-feels"* (Sela-Smith 85). This resistance came out of fear around revisiting some of my childhood and so the question became, not only was I willing to make that journey but also, could I truly surrender to the painful feelings of the experience itself? Even the thought was a bit terrifying. I could remember past feelings associated with the memories but intuitively I knew I had to commit to allowing the "I who feels" (Sela-Smith 74) rather than the, "I who observes" to engage in the experience. Sela-Smith distinguishes these two concepts and her major critique of Moustakas' methodology was that it was not possible to stay in the "feeling I" (74). When I stayed in the "feeling I," I felt a sense of panic in knowing there would be no turning back. There were no "hypotheses or expectations regarding outcomes, no hope to confirm or refute a proposition. There was no attempt to isolate variables or observe the effects one set of variables has on other variables within the research" (Sela-Smith 83). There was just my internal self and my experiences. It was frightening. Would I be able to stay the course or would this be just another failure? Shades of my insecurities and fear of failure from my past overshadowed my desire to work through the resistance that I knew would be there. When this resistance became so strong that I felt as though I was choking and my breathing became restricted would I be able to overcome it and complete the journey? Could I move through the resistance and allow complete surrender? The journey itself would answer these questions.

In the final analysis my methodology drew on the wisdom of both Moustakas and Sela-Smith. I brought into the research my life, my experiences and some deep seated preconceived ideas based on tacit knowledge being "the deep structure that contains the unique perceptions, feelings, intuitions, beliefs, and judgments housed in the internal frame of reference of a person that governs behavior and determines how we interpret experience" (Moustakas 32). Tacit knowledge is implied or understood knowledge from within in which we just *know* that we know something without understanding how or why we know it. Sela-Smith believes that tacit knowledge can be flawed (61), and that since it can be flawed then it can also be changed as transformation takes place in the research process. A child touches the burner of the stove and burns her hand. In the future she instinctively, through tacit knowledge, *knows* the stove is hot whether or not the burner is on. Sela-Smith makes the point that the key to healing or change is in accessing the tacit structure through feelings. I cannot experience healing by talking about the feelings; I must enter into them and "feel" them.

In the <u>initial engagement</u> phase my question arose out of my intense fascination with the connection between healing and story. In my ministry as staff chaplain I listen to the stories of others on a daily basis and witness healing at various levels in peoples' lives. Initially it was my intent to study the experiences of others and look at an external connection. I became keenly aware that there were stories hidden in the recesses of my memory and my question germinated in my soul. The "crucial process" of "focusing on a topic" (Moustakas 39) was one in which I wrestled with the question and finally it crystallized. Heuristics invited me to explore my own stories and the self-encounter of those junctures of time in the experiences in my life as they cried out to be explored in a way that sought to discover that connection between my healing and my story. I knew intuitively that my own stories and my own inner healing journey needed to be the focus of my study. This was another crucial process and part of "collecting the data" (Moustakas 39) for my research.

The <u>immersion phase</u> then invited me to that process of "concentrated gazing" (Moustakas 39) in which I step back in time and identify with the focus of inquiry by becoming one with my question. I had to let the question speak to me, to inform me as part of the "crucial process ... methods of preparing and collecting ... data" (Moustakas 39). The following diagram perhaps best reflects the process as I moved back and forth between the various stages. The only story that I wrote completely at one sitting, although I rewrote it many times, was "Through the Eyes of a Child." The others I wrote simultaneously and in bites and pieces. As the diagram indicates the process was back and forth from one stage to another. The circles are numbered simply as a way of following the process.

Data Gathering and Reflection Process

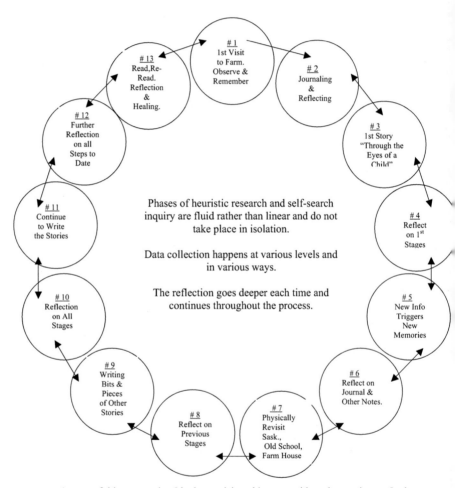

As part of this preparation I had to revisit and interact with each experience. In the words of Michael Maley, Ph.D., I had to "live in the Question," which meant I needed to "be open to personal transformations in which formlessness has been experienced and integrated into the psyche" (Maley 179). (This idea may have come from the work of nineteenth-century poet, Rainer Maria Rilke.) In my mind I had to allow the memories of each experience to flood my being. I truly began to live the question and everything in my life spoke of healing and story. My radio, my pastor, my colleagues all seemed to be reading my mind and knowing what I needed to hear at any particular moment. I return to the scene of each of the experiences in chapter four. I revisit the family farm with my daughter and grandson and subsequently on my own. I visit the home of my grandparents and explore the old dilapidated house where no one had lived for years. I go to the farm where I lived until I was three years old. I visit the old school house and walk in the yard. I go to Thompson, Manitoba to the cemetery and spend time at my husband's grave. I drive past the house we built. I even stop and knock on the door and speak to the man who lives there now. On the return trip I stop along the highway at the exact spot where the accident happened. I get out and sit on the bank of the river and remember and cry. I go to Leney, Saskatchewan to the cemetery where both of my parents and my brother are buried. I spend one winter month at a retreat center where I walk for hours along the shore of the lake. I find solitude in the long drives to Saskatchewan and back, and on the daily commute back and forth between Edmonton and Red Deer. At times I walk with my sister and we share our memories, the similarities and the differences in our growing up years. I have often kept a journal but now it becomes more intentional. I write constantly. I write as I travel, even pulling over on the side of the road when a voice inside my head or a voice on my radio speaks to me. I begin to take a tape recorder with me in my car so I can record thoughts, feelings and memories. I am aware that the preparation and the data collection are overlapping. It is hard to tell where one ends and the other begins as I write my stories, read them, rewrite them, read them again and then rewrite them again.

It is in this phase that the "crucial process" of "organizing" and beginning the process of "analyzing" (Moustakas 39) my discoveries and newfound knowledge come into play. Sela-Smith's methodology challenged me to stay in the moment, to stay present to the feelings and to surrender to the entire process. "*Finally, there must be an acceptance of surrender that opens to transformation that can impact the individual, society, and all of humankind*" (Sela-Smith 85). Sela-Smith's interpretation of heuristics intrigued me, frightened me and challenged me to look at my own experience of inner healing in ways that I had not previously allowed myself to do. I had to be willing to feel at the deepest level of my inner being. I had to be vulnerable and transparent throughout the process. The surrender has been difficult. There were memories that I did not want to dredge up. But as I stepped back for a period of incubation, (Moustakas 28) to reflect on the experiences and allow them to permeate my entire being this surrender slowly became a reality. At this point I could truly appreciate the words of Rilke, as cited by Henry Nouwen,

> Be patient towards all that is unsolved in your heart. And try to love the
> questions themselves … Do not now seek answers which cannot be given you
> because you would not be able to live them. And the point is to love
> everything. *Live* the questions now. Perhaps you will then gradually, without
> noticing it, live along some distant day into the answer (Nouwen 41).

Being patient and allowing myself to just be in the moment and in the question calls me to live and love the question—the answers will take care of themselves. In the patience and the quiet the answers will come. They cannot be forced. And so I sat alone with my inner child. I sat, in memory, with my mom and I sat with my poetry and let it speak to me. I walked in my memory with my dad and came to understand his life and was able to forgive his transgressions and accept him for who he was. I was, however, unable to be with my brother, even in my memory. The awareness of that was painful but healthy. There are opportunities for healing to continue in my life. Incubation allowed for maturation and the informing of self and then ultimately moved to illuminate my understanding.

Illumination (Moustakas 29) occurs when the unconscious awareness becomes conscious and new understandings come to the forefront. The flawed tacit knowledge of my formative years underwent transformation as my worldview shifted Sometimes illumination happened for me as I was reliving the experience. Spending joyous time with my grandson on the family farm triggered a shift in perception and the fullness of my childhood memories was restored. Life's experiences spoke to me in new and unexpected ways and transformation took place. My perception changed as I was able to seeing the bigger picture.

The explication phase (Moustakas 30-31) called me to "examine various layers of meaning that have been disclosed" (Sela-Smith 68). The "crucial processes of analyzing and synthesizing data" (Moustakas 39), came into play as I read my stories and began to reframe the stories in reflection. In this process of reflection I allowed new discovery to be revealed. It is here that I became aware of the various levels of healing that are possible through story. I explored all aspects of the connection as I sought to discover the experience of healing as revealed through story. Was there healing in the writing of the story, revisiting the experience and attempting to move back into the feelings of the experience, or in the telling or sharing of the story? Perhaps there was healing in the listening as I reread my stories, stepped back and listened as though I were hearing them for the first time. Which aspects of story fostered healing? This is all part of my heuristic reflection chapter. I attempted to pay particular attention to the feelings, thoughts, beliefs and judgments of my lived experience as I wrote and reflected on those experiences.

Moustakas' final phase is <u>creative synthesis</u> (31). This phase incorporates the "crucial process of synthesizing data" (Moustakas 39), which allows the new story to evolve out of the entire process through reflection on the overall experience of writing and sharing my personal journey to inner healing. My personal transformation must be evident to my readers as they experience my story.

The final step in my methodology was to look at the validity of the entire process. According to Moustakas, "The question of validity is one of meaning" (Moustakas 32). Validation is found in the authenticity of my own experience as the researcher. This was not an easy task for it demanded both transparency and vulnerability. Self-dialogue and self-honesty both required deep soul searching in efforts to reveal the depth of the experience from the inner most part of my being. It was most important for me to be attentive and present to my feelings and my dialogue with those feelings in the realization that "to report a feeling is not the same as dialoguing with the feeling" (Sela-Smith 69). Diligence was required on my part as I undertook the heuristic inquiry of reflecting, sifting, exploring and judging both relevance and meaning so as to accurately depict not only the experience but also the internal shift in self discovery and understanding as "I am actively awakening and transforming my own self" (Moustakas 13).

According to Sela-Smith,

> Validity of the research is established by surrendering to the process that is pushing itself into the consciousness of the researcher, allowing the process to unfold and then noticing results in expansion of self-awareness, deepening of self-understanding, and of self-transformation that others can experience in the 'story' (79).

Surrendering to the experience was somewhat like giving birth. It was difficult but once the process started there was no turning back. I encountered resistance and pain, but amidst the pangs of birthing, the beauty of a new creation pushed itself into being. In awe I stepped back and realized my world had changed.

An important aspect of validation throughout my process came as I shared my stories with my sisters. Validation came from sharing my stories and discovering that some of my sisters were willing and able to listen to my stories and interact with me through the shared experiences of having grown up in an alcoholic household. Validation also came through the inability of one of my sisters to listen to my experiences or to share her experiences with us. Her denial confirmed and validated my experiences and was part of my growth and new understanding. Each of us had our own experiences, some were shared and others were unique but alcoholism and dysfunction were part of the shared reality that validated my experiences.

Validation has two layers. Internal validation comes through personal growth, transformation and healing revealed through reflection. External validation comes as I hold my experience in dialogue with the literature on healing and writers such as, Buechner, Desalvo, Graham, Lewis and Pelzer, all of whom echo my experiences in their work, validate my story. Just as we know the Bible is true when it tells our own story, similarly, my readers know my story is true when their lives and mine reflect each other. Our experiences are unique but our judgments coincide.

Chapter Summary

In summary it is important to recognize the works of both Moustakas and Sela-Smith. The combination of their methodologies gave me the tools I needed to undertake a heuristic self-search inquiry in which I sought to gain new insights and understanding through researching my question, "What is the experience of healing as revealed through story?"

Both Moustakas and Sela-Smith agreed upon these six phases of heuristic/self-search inquiry: the initial engagement, immersion, incubation, illumination, explication and creative synthesis. I appreciated Sela-Smith's divergence from Moustakas with her emphasis on the self or the "I-who-feels," the resistance to being in the feelings and the focus on internal search. My research was very much an inner healing journey in which Sela-Smith's concepts were an important aspect of my journey. There are similarities with Moustakas' concepts and processes and Sela-Smith's key components. Moustakas identified: identifying the focus of inquiry; self dialogue; tacit knowledge; intuition; indwelling; and focusing and internal frame of reference (15-27), while Sela-Smith highlighted six key components which were important to her self-search inquiry: the researcher must have experienced what is identified as being researched; the researcher makes reference to some intense or passionate concern that causes the investigator to reach inward for tacit awareness and knowledge; the researcher indicates surrender to the question has taken place (living, waking, sleeping, and dreaming the question); self-dialogue, not simply a one-way reporting of thoughts or feelings is evidenced, (to report a feeling is not the same as dialoguing with the feeling); the search is a self-search; and there is evidence that transformation has taken place (69).

In addition Moustakas identified three crucial processes: concentrated gazing, focusing on the topic or formulation of the question and methods of preparing, collecting, organizing, analyzing and synthesizing data (39). Sela-Smith concluded that the applications of heuristic research are threefold; recognition of the value of self-search inquiry and a return to the internal perspective, acknowledgement of resistance to feeling in the reconnection with the *I-who-feels,* and acceptance of surrender that opens to transformation (85).

These phases, concepts, crucial processes, key components and threefold application, of these two noted proponents of heuristics, along with a process of validation, laid the foundation for my work and allowed me the flexibility needed to complete my research.

It is also important to recognize that part of my methodology was the inclusion of an ethicist. This was a variance from the methodologies of either Moustakas or Sela-Smith but I deemed it to be necessary because of the extremely personal nature of my research. Ethical considerations and my journey with Dr. Davis Mathias, as ethicist, are dealt with in detail in chapter three.

CHAPTER THREE

ETHICAL CONSIDERATIONS

Ethics, as defined by *A Handbook of Health Ethics*, prepared by a multi-disciplinary committee at the Bioethics Centre at The University of Alberta, states succinctly what we mean by ethics.

> Ethics is concerned with the norms of right and wrong, and of "ought"' and "ought not", and in respect to values and behaviours between persons. Our ethical decisions involve reasoning and emotions. Our ethical decisions take into account not only the facts but also what is important, the sacrifices we may need to make, and how our choices affect those around us (2).

Determining those norms of right and wrong is not easy. The realization that recording my stories would, of necessity involve other family members caused me to consider possible ethical concerns that might arise and then take the necessary steps to minimize negative effects. My major ethical concern, as I began my heuristic research/self-search inquiry, arose around the realization that my stories were not mine alone. I shared life with a family of eleven siblings, two parents and numerous relatives, neighbors and friends. Each one was a part of my story just as I was part of theirs. I needed to examine and determine, whether these stories would bring any measure of harm to those who were part of my stories, including myself. Secondly, during the reflection process of this dissertation, the possibility of re- traumatizing myself became a reality. A third consideration was to look at my need to tell the stories and a fourth was to weigh just how much detail was required and for what purpose. I had to be true to the experience and to myself as I approached my writing in an ethical manner that reflected my Christian values.

My internal struggles led me to approach the HREB (Health Research Ethics Board) to determine if I was required to present a proposal to them. They indicated that since I was not interviewing others I did not need to meet that requirement. I next approached my committee and presented my ethical concerns to them. They reminded me that, "the truth shall set you free" (John 8:32). The importance was to tell the stories as they related to my own healing and to recognize and acknowledge that it was not my intent to cause discomfort or harm to anyone by disclosure of my experiences. While this partially helped to put my mind at ease there was still an element of dis-ease as I started to write.

For my own peace of mind I contacted a Christian moral ethicist, Dr. Rebecca Davis Mathias. Dr. Davis Mathias is an ethicist with Caritas Health Group and St. Joseph's Auxiliary Hospital. She is assistant professor at St. Joseph's College, University of Alberta, where she teaches, among other things, Bioethics, Advanced Bioethics, Business Ethics, and Social Justice. Initially the two of us met for a period of two hours during which time I outlined the direction my dissertation was taking and expressed my concerns with regards to the ethical considerations presented previously. Dr. Davis Mathias agreed to journey with me as an ethicist and to guide my dissertation. She read my stories from an ethical standpoint and highlighted any areas that appeared to present problems. At one particular point in one of my stories, she suggested that rather than naming one of my brothers, I should protect his identity by simply writing "my brother." This did not change the context or meaning and yet protected his identity and respected his right to privacy and the principle of confidentiality. I concurred with this and made that change. Together we looked at other ethical concerns such as disclosure, wording, privacy, respect, interpretation and boundaries.

We addressed those concerns in ways that allowed for integrity in the process while still maintaining authenticity and transparency.

Dr. Davis Mathias directed me to the Health Ethics Guide put together by the Catholic Health Association of Canada. It made sense to me that since I utilize this guide in my ministry on a daily basis, I should also use its wisdom as I struggled with ethical concerns in writing my own inner healing journey. The fundamental values of respecting the dignity of every human person and the interconnectedness of every human being guided our discussions and my writings as I wrote of my father's alcoholism and the resulting abuse while looking forward to the common good that could result. Working through the process allowed me to be true to my experience and voice what I needed to say without transgressing confidentiality of my father's story.

Dr. Davis Mathias and I looked at the entire process of ethical discernment to discover which elements were applicable to my particular concerns. The guide is written for the medical communities but,

> complements other initiatives in the church's (Roman Catholic) healing ministry, such as spiritual/religious care, organizational mission and values integration, ethics committees and centers, and parish based ministry/nursing, through which caregivers are becoming more aware of the broader aspects of their healing ministry (ix).

These Christian moral values and principles extend beyond denominational or faith tradition boundaries and contribute wisdom to ethical decision making in society as a whole. They have transference capacity that is easily adaptable to my life in general and more specifically to the heuristic research/self search inquiry of this dissertation.

The framework for ethical discernment, re-printed from the *Health Ethics Guide*

(81), summarizing the values and principles adhered to by the Catholic Health Association of Canada, is capsulated in a simple diagram. I was a member of the Caritas Ethics Committee for a couple of years and found opportunity to test both the methods and the positions outlined in the booklet. The purpose of the guide is to facilitate sound ethical reflection that leads to informed decision-making. The Christian moral values and principles apply equally to ministry and personal life through the process for ethical discernment that can easily be adapted for me as I work through the ethical concerns that arise as I write.

A Framework for Ethical Discernment

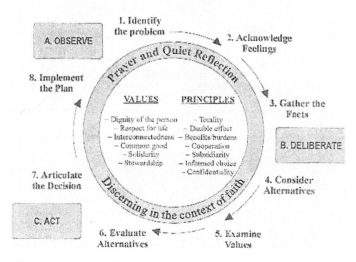

"Christian ethical reasoning is based upon a world-view contained in the gospel ... and gives rise to values and principles that direct ethical decision making"(11). The fundamental values and principles are shown in the diagram above reprinted with permission.

The works and writings of others have convinced me that it is not only ethically correct, but also ethically responsible for me to write, share and reflect on my own experiences. The stories need to be told, not only for my own healing and growth but also for the healing and growth of others.

Natasha Bedingfield in her debut disc's title cut, "Unwritten" encourages her listeners to "Release your inhibitions." That message is compelling as I tell my story. But the words of Charlie Martin, columnist for the *Prairie Messenger*, as he reflects on the words of Bedingfield, tell us that,

> Inhibitions that caution you not to harm yourself or others or to break a relationship with God are helpful. But don't diminish what your life can be through narrow or negative thinking. Instead, focus on the grandest vision you can imagine. See yourself creating a positive difference with your life. Write your story in ways that help the rest of us become better (10).

I believe both Bedingfield and Martin were speaking more of how we live our lives in the creation of our story, but for me these words of advice are equally as important in the revisiting and telling our stories.

Richard Gula writes, "while we are certainly called to do what is right as Christians, we are first of all called to be loving persons in the imitation of Christ … who we are matters morally" (7). I needed to consider what was right for me as a Christian and could I be both right and loving in delving into and exposing family secrets? So, ethically and morally, what is demanded of me as a follower of Christ? Years ago I read Charles Sheldon's, *In His Steps,* originally written in 1896, in which an entire community determined to live their lives asking the question, "What would Jesus do?" before making any major decisions. The idea appealed to me and subsequently I tried to live my life asking that question. As I recently read Gula's words I was reminded of Sheldon's book and now asked myself that question in regards to writing my healing journey. What would Christ do? How much of my journey was it necessary to tell and what was better left unsaid? Ethically I had to look at why I was doing what I was doing. Was it simply for my own satisfaction or was there a greater good? In looking at this with Davis Mathias and my committee, I recognized that the greater good is perhaps revealed through my courage to relive and then to share my personal healing journey in the hopes that doing so might be the catalyst to encourage others to undertake the initiative to explore their own healing journey. We do not travel this road of life alone and while our experiences are unique they are not so different. The truth that sets us free, I believe, is in Christ Jesus.

> The crucial insight and realization, which opens up a whole new dimension of personal growth, is this: Something in me—my attitudes, my vision of reality—determines all my actions and reactions, both emotional and behavioral. Something in me is writing the story of my life, making it sad and sorrowful or glad and peaceful. Something in me will ultimately make the venture of my life a success or a failure. The sooner I acknowledge this, taking responsibility for my actions and reactions, the faster I will move toward my destiny; the fullness of life and peace. This fullness of life and peace is our legacy from the Lord (John Powell, S. J. 15).

In the above quotation, Powell speaks to the perception we hold of ourselves and the limitations placed on the ability to live our life to that fullest built-in potential God intended for us to achieve.

Sources that have given me strength for the journey have been read and reread in preparation for this doctoral work. As I reread Powell's words I realized that it was and is impossible for me to live life to my fullest potential without facing the reality of my painful memories and moving in healing to that wholeness referred to by Maddix and Soles (2003).

Chapter Summary

As I introduced the issues I identified the major ethical concerns I faced in undertaking this dissertation:

1. Concern over the possibility of harm to family and others

2. The possibility of re-traumatizing myself

3. What was my need to tell my stories?

4. How much detail was required?

After identifying these concerns I approached the HREB to ascertain that I was following proper protocol. I sought out an ethicist to journey with me as I explored what was ethically correct and then went to the *Health Ethics Guide* for direction and insight. There were numerous points along the journey in which, as part of my ethical discernment I looked at those principles and values within the framework set out in the guide and questioned why I was doing what I was doing? Davis Mathias was a great asset as she helped me to discern what was necessary and what was not. I needed to respect my family and yet at the same time claim my reality in the knowledge that perhaps there was a greater good.

As I moved into the reflection stage the questions were still there:

1. How much needed to be revealed?

2. To what extent did I need to risk exposing myself, and others, simply because they happened to be part of my inner circle?

3. Was it sufficient to have made the journey?

4. Does every sordid detail have to be included as part of my story?

5. Do I risk re-traumatizing myself in the journey?

6. Which part of this process is healthy and is any part of it unhealthy?

I attempted to respond to the questions and find that balance, which allowed me to respect others and still permit my own healing journey to continue as I recognized that I am not the same person who lived those experiences. I have changed.

The principles and morals of Christian ethics served as guideposts throughout the entire process as I entered into relationship with myself, and others who were involved in my experiences. As I wrote, I attempted, as much as possible, to maintain a sense of dignity and respect while promoting justice and fostering truth. Justice comes in revealing the truth and then allowing it to set us free. From John's Gospel we have the assurance that there is freedom in truth (John 8:32). That was the assurance I sought as I gave myself permission to write what I needed to write. The following chapter introduces the reader to four such stories from the pages of my life.

CHAPTER FOUR

STRAIGHT FROM MY HEART

Gene Fowler said, "Writing is easy; all you do is sit staring at a blank sheet of paper until the drops of blood form on your forehead" (qtd. in Bartlett 678).

I have experienced firsthand staring at a blank sheet of paper. I have felt the drops of blood although my mirror denied their existence. It is after the drops of blood ooze from the depths of my inner being, from my very soul, that the lifelines intertwined as my stories cry out from the pit of my gut to be heard.

These are my stories. They are from the heart and soul of my life. They are from the recesses of my memory. They are stories of pain and of healing, of sorrow and of joy. The joy comes in knowing that I am no longer stuck in that space in my life. There have been moments of significant transition and growth as I moved on and discovered that I am indeed on that journey towards wholeness that Maddix and Soles address. The healing journey does not end because life itself is a journey that is full of surprises. It is comprised of mountaintop experiences and times of being in the shadow of the valley of death. If we did not have the valley experiences we would not recognize the mountaintop experiences. Each has its own reward. I am who I am because of my lived experiences, which I share with you willingly and only ask that you tread lightly. You are reading my soul.

Through the Eyes of a Child

"Come Grams—let's vestigate—let's vestigate"

Matheau ran off ahead, his wide blue eyes taking in the expanse of the farmyard and coming to focus on the dilapidated old barn. Once before he and his mom had lived in a place in which there was an old building with a loft and Matheau loved the loft. He had decided the barn would be the first object for his "vestigation." Perhaps there would be a loft for him to play in. The old barn tweaked his six-year old curiosity.

The two of us scrambled through the foot-high broom grass and prairie thistle that stretched from the farmyard to the barnyard. The barn seemed somehow fragile, not quite as majestic as it had once been. It tilted precariously off center threatening to collapse if a strong north winter wind blew, as it was prone to do in this part of Saskatchewan. But it was summer time and that day we basked in the heat of the sun. At one time the barn was painted crimson red and stood straight and proud. It seemed to tell the entire world that it was home for the Herefords, the Angus, the stallions and the mares.

On that hot summer day the emptiness seemed to echo the memories of yesteryear and that old barn seemed to come alive as we wandered through the old stalls and finally up to the loft. The dusty old straw and the pungent smell of manure permeated the place with a fragrance that brought the barn back to life. The sound was that of eerie quiet that seemed to invite us to venture in. The loft was empty except for binder twine ropes that hung from the ceiling and I could picture Dad and Grandpa swinging the straw bales and piling them high as they stored up the hay for the winter's feed. Matheau excitedly grabbed a rope and started to swing.

"Oh, Grams, this is fun. I like it here. Are you and Grandpa going to live here with us?"

"No, Matheau, we're not –but I used to live here. This is where Grams grew up."

The memories came flooding back. I had not been back to the farm, other than for brief visits, for a number of years. The farm had been vacant for about six years since my brother Victor moved into North Battleford. The entire district was nearly deserted with most of the farmers living in nearby towns or in the city and choosing to farm from a distance. As I drove to the farm earlier that weekend there was a hollowness that seemed to echo the emptiness of the deserted farmhouses that dotted the landscape. Tweedyside district, which was our district, at one time bustled with activity. It even had a school and a hall. I went to that country school for my elementary schooling. The local hall hosted many community events, such as Christmas concerts (a thing of the past) and family dances, which always started out to be so much fun. I could conjure up in my mind the sound of Longworths' orchestra playing the old waltzes and the Fox trot. Uncle Ulysse called many a square dance and the rafters shook with merriment. I learned to dance standing on my dad's feet and moving with him to the music. Everyone danced at the country-dances and when the littlest ones tired out the coats would be spread out along the wall and soon there were children asleep amidst the music and laughter. You could bet money and your odds would be much better than any lottery today (it was a sure thing) that before the evening came to an end the men would get drunk and the brawls would start. There didn't need to be a reason. Neighbor would fight against neighbor and brother against brother while the women and children stayed out of the way as much as possible. Numerous times, too numerous to count, as we returned home Dad would be shouting. His rhetoric went something like, "That's it—

we'll have nothing more to do with the Mainland's (my mom's sister and brother-in-law) or the Scott's (our godparents) or the Mairs (neighbors) or any other neighbor who happened to be on the wrong end of Dad's anger or his fists. "Don't you be phoning them either." He would admonish my mom. And we were never again to speak to whoever had been on the other end of the fight on that particular night. But sure as the sun would come up, Monday morning would role around and we'd all be off to school together and Mom and Aunty Jean would be chatting on the phone as usual. Sometimes they would wait until the men had gone to the field for the day but then after a day or so all would be back to "normal" whatever that was. This scenario played over and over again and was part of my childhood.

My love/hate relationships flourished amidst family violence and community violence that seemed to be accepted as the norm. That really did something to my psyche and had a life-long affect on how I view alcohol and violence. This farm represented all of that to me.

And now my daughter and her son were moving here to live. My daughter Starla was a single mom who always loved animals and the great outdoors. When she was young, about in grade two, she brought home a white mouse hoping to keep it as a pet. When she was very young I would catch her playing with the caterpillars on the sidewalk. She'd put one on her hand and watch it climb up her arm. She was fascinated with nature and so it should not have been a surprise to me that she would jump at the opportunity to be a hobby farmer or at least live on a farm. Sometimes I asked myself, "Is she really my daughter?" I, who am allergic to animals and am truly a city person, have this daughter so different from myself. She is truly her own person and I am so proud of her. She had recently rented the farmhouse and the surrounding yard from her Uncle Victor. This particular weekend was moving weekend and I was helping them move and cleanup the yard.

I tried to hide my feelings without knowing exactly what those feelings were as my daughter told me that she and Matheau were going to rent the farm and live there. As a youngster I had hated that farm, at times with every fiber of my being. We were the poor Whitfield's and as if being poor wasn't punishment enough, my father was an alcoholic. "My daddy was a farmer and all he ever raised was us" is a line from an old country and western song "Po' Folks." I listened to the original rendition as a kid and was sure it had been written specifically for our family. But that song had some lines that didn't always fit at our household. "We'd patch the cracks and set the table with love." Oh, Mom tried and I suppose even Dad did in his own way. Who knows which came first, the drinking or the poverty? Did the poverty influence the drinking or did the drinking create the poverty? I suppose the question is rhetorical and a little like asking, which came first the chicken or the egg? I only know that for me living in our household seemed to be a living hell. I could not wait to get away from that place. And here I was helping my daughter and her son to move to this God forsaken place.

Alcoholism is a strange disease that like any other addiction affects the entire family. There is some evidence that there is a genetic disposition towards it and I grew up believing that to be true. Although my grandfather never admitted it I'm convinced he was an alcoholic just like his son and as they grew up, some of my brothers became alcoholics. I was afraid I would *catch it* and vowed that I would never be like them. Alcohol had a strange power over our household and I didn't like it one bit.

I was always told I had a chip on my shoulder and I believe I did. I spent much of my life proving I was as good as anyone else (maybe even just a little better), which was a hard concept for me to grasp. It's hard to believe in yourself when you wear hand-me-down clothes and sometimes can't even find a brush or a comb and "there's a whole lotta people looking down their noses at me, cause I didn't come from a wealthy family." The words were those of Bill Anderson but I had a sense he just sang the song while I lived it. There were twelve of us and with Mom and Dad we totaled fourteen. It wasn't easy growing up in a family of twelve kids on ¼ section of land. I remember joking with Mom and telling her that they should have quit after I was born. As a teenager I was embarrassed that my mom was always pregnant. I decided I would never get married and certainly would never have any kids. I didn't want to be like Mom. It took having my own children and grandchildren to understand the magnitude of the dreams my mother gave up for us.

Grandma and grandpa had lived on this farm before us and when they retired to Vancouver we moved from an even poorer farmhouse to this one. At the old farmhouse, called the Fishback place (I guess Fishbacks lived there before we did) there were eight of us living in three small rooms. I have vague memories of life there but then I was only three when we moved to our "new" home. We had Saskatoon berries, raspberries and strawberries at the old place. Oh, and we had garter snakes and other crawly things. I remember one bright colored garter snake that we captured and put down the well to drown it. It must have been six feet long. (Through the eyes of a child.) I thought it was a rattlesnake, if I even knew what they were. I remember going with Mom to pick the berries. We had lots of fruit in those days and Saskatoons became, and remain, my very favorite.

At the new place at least we had more room, which was kind of necessary because just as we moved, Mom brought home another new baby. It seems there was always a new baby at our house.

Our new house was rather large in comparison to the former one. It had an upstairs that Grandpa fixed up to be four bedrooms. Grandpa was a carpenter. He built this house when he and grandma came from England to settle on the Saskatchewan prairies. On the main floor was a kitchen and multipurpose room. The kitchen had a bay window and it felt good to sit there in the sunshine, watch Mom bake and savor the smell of hot apple pie or fresh bread. Mom was an excellent cook and we certainly never went hungry.

The bathroom was called the outhouse and was a short walk from the house. For baths we hauled water from the spring and heated it on our coal and wood stove. The younger children got to bath first and I guess they were the cleanest because we older ones had to bath in the same water.

The memories are all jumbled up. My mind's eye envisions grandpa coming, as he did every seedtime and harvest-time. He traveled by train and it was usually late at night when he arrived and we would get to stay up late to greet him and receive the little gifts he always brought with him. There was such excitement. But then the excitement wore off as the weekend rolled around and Dad and Grandpa would head off to town and the beer parlor. They'd close down the pub and the inevitable would happen. Dad and Grandpa Charlie, which is what we called him most of the time, would get into an argument about something that really didn't matter much except to them in their drunken stupors and the fight would be on. In those days we had the old phone that hung on the wall. The type that you rang three long and two short and all the neighbors could listen in because you were on what they called a party line. I have vivid memories of that phone being torn off the wall as Mom tried to make a phone call. Somehow I had a sense that Mom, like us kids, was afraid that one of them might get killed the way they went at each other. To tell the truth I'm rather surprised they both survived all those battles. Sometimes it would be a relief to see Grandpa go back to Vancouver. But the weekends still came and went.

I was ashamed to have my friends come to my house. I hated my father when he got drunk and caused such a scene. I never knew what my father would do if he came home in a rage. Sometimes just the stupid things, like taking a piss off the back step. (Remember we lived in the country.) Sometimes things were more violent, things like laying a beating on my brother or throwing a chair at him and leaving that huge hole in the wall. Mom was leaving many times but I suppose she never knew what she would do if she left and how would she support the family? Which kids would she take and which would stay with Dad? My mind has an image of my older sister and I standing with Mom at the front door, suitcases in hand, while the boys and Dad stood on the other side of the room. There was lots of yelling going on and I don't recall the words but eventually the suitcases got unpacked and put away. We didn't leave.

I hated that farm, that place where I grew up. But what was it I really hated? And was hatred really the appropriate word? Perhaps the appropriate word was abhorred, which "implies a deep, often shuddering repugnance" (Webster's Collegiate Dictionary 44). That particular definition seems to fit what I felt.

As Matheau and I explored the old farm and laughed and ran together, memories of gentler times seeped into my memory. The cement exterior of my mind seemed to have cracked, as had the foundation of the old barn.

The house didn't much resemble the farmhouse of my childhood. My brother victor had maintained the framework and built around it to what today was a beautiful sprawling ranch house. But farming had not been kind to him and he had moved to North Battleford to make a living. And so the ranch house was neglected and looked much older than it should. The years of vacancy and the weather had not been kind. It needed some tender loving care and my daughter thought she could provide that. A few months earlier Starla and I had journeyed to Saskatchewan for a family funeral and she had asked if we could go out to the old farm. I think she already had in mind that she wanted to live there although what it was that beckoned her was beyond my comprehension.

Matheau and I had such fun as we continued to explore. "Mom, come join us" called Matheau as we walked through the yard past the house. "Okay, be right there." Starla put aside what she was doing and hurried to join us. After the barn we "vestigated" the creek bed and ran down to where the old road used to be and I found myself telling Matheau of the fun times I had experienced here as a child.

"Matheau, see this spring. We hauled our drinking water from here. Feel it—it's ice cold even when it's hot outside. That's because the spring that feeds the well runs under the ground and the ground keeps it cold."

"Wow, that's cold." Matheau ran further down along side the stream. "Can I take my shoes off and go in the water."

"Sure, if it's okay with your mom."

Starla nodded her agreement and Matheau squealed as the icy water closed in around his toes and then his ankles as he ventured deeper.

"Matheau, can you imagine not having hot and cold running water like we have today? We carried water up to the house in pails and then heated it in buckets on the stove." It seemed as though time stood still or perhaps took a step backwards that day. Matheau, a typical six-year-old, soon tired of the water and was anxious to explore further. We wandered over to a valley like area surrounded by trees and just beside the spring. "This area is where my mom would take us children for a picnic." I told Matheau and Starla. "She'd pack a picnic basket, spread out a blanket and we would pretend we were on holidays. Mom would sometimes bring her guitar. We'd sit on the blanket, listen to Mom play and we'd have a sing along. Then we'd have our picnic lunch and then play some games like hide and seek while Mom sat and watched us. We weren't very old then. I probably wasn't any older than you are now. Can you imagine eating dandelions? My mom used to make salads out of them. I don't really remember what they tasted like and I'm not sure I liked them much but they were part of the picnic." I remembered that Mom improvised a lot and probably the dandelion salads were served at those times when we didn't have much else for a salad. Matheau seemed content to simply enjoy the vast open space of the farm and to listen to the tales I, his grams, told him of my childhood memories.

Other memories came forward to claim their space. Christmas Eve was a special time at our house and I remember it fondly. The Mainland's always came to our house Christmas Eve. Dad and Uncle Sid would hitch up the horses to the sleigh or the buggy and we would all pile in to go Christmas Caroling throughout the neighborhood. It was such fun. The horses were decked out in bells and we'd pull in to the neighbors' yards and sing a couple of carols before gleefully going off to the next yard. At the end of the evening it was back to our house for a treat of Japanese oranges and pop. Dad would always find the money to buy a couple of wooden crates of glass-bottled pop and those special Christmas oranges. My favorite pop was 7-up and on this night you got to pick your favorite.

A memory that is both pleasant and disturbing is of Mom sitting at her sewing machine all night sewing or remodeling clothes for us. That memory reminds me of how much our mother loved us and tried to erase the poverty we lived in. At those times I would feel a little ashamed of myself for hating who we were. But I dreamed of escaping the farm. Somehow I felt trapped there and I wanted to be far, far away.

I wanted to be far away from the fighting, from Dad's temper; from feeling I had to stick up for my brother who always seemed to be the object of Dad's anger. I wanted to escape to a better life, far, far away from our rundown shack, from the constant bickering of my parents, from the piles of dirty laundry and the unkempt house, from the worn out linoleum and the penury that seemed to follow me everywhere.

Matheau and I, accompanied by Starla, continued to "vestigate" and then wandered back to the house. The grass and weeds in the yard were thick and long. Uncle Victor had loaned Starla his small tractor with a mower blade for the cleanup. While she and Matheau unpacked in the house I undertook to attack the yard. For the next couple of hours I rode the tractor, which was something I never got to do on the farm. I never got to drive anything except the horses. I grew up in a very patriarchal family where the boys were boys and girls were girls and there was no crossing of the lines of responsibility. The boys worked outside on the land with Dad while the girls were expected to do the girl things like cook, scrub and wash the clothes. I remember when I turned sixteen I asked Dad if he would teach me to drive. Mom never had a license and I only remember her driving once. She needed to go into town and Dad was out in the field. She started up the old Model A—chug, chug, jerk,

jerk, and off we went—right into the chicken fence. Chickens were squawking and running every which way. That was the end of Mom's driving. "I didn't teach the boys to drive— they just drove." Dad informed me. I asked for the keys to the truck. Dad put his hand in his pocket, pulled out the keys, looked at them and without a word put them back in his pocket and turned away. So much for my learning to drive! I learned to drive after I left home.

But today I could ride the tractor. As the tractor went round and round; as both grass and weeds disappeared, so too did the heartache, hatred, resentment and bitter memories. I was at peace with the farm at last. This farm was part of me. My roots were here and I had come home—not on my terms but on Matheau's.

The Teenage Years

"There's been an accident. Come Quickly!!" The words were spoken to my parents, but the entire household was awakened and abuzz. Thirteen-year-old Gordon, from a neighboring farm, had crawled to his parents' home, bleeding profusely and badly injured. The words his parents heard were the same words that now echoed throughout our household.

My brother Dick and I exchanged glances. "Let's go," he said. My memories are blurred. I don't remember how we went the mile and a half down the road to where the twisted wreck, that once was a half-ton truck, lay in the ditch. I do remember seeing the body of our eldest brother, Bill, lying in a pool of his own blood on the roadway. "Go home!" Dad barked at us as he saw us standing there. The terrible horror of what was unfolding grabbed at my heart.

In stunned silence we returned home and waited, staring at the closed door; waiting for it to open and for Mom and Dad to confirm our worst nightmare.

"Bill's dead." Mom sobbed and collapsed as she came in the door. Bill was working for a neighboring farmer, helping with the late fall work. He, accompanied by the neighbor's son, had gone into town and had obviously been drinking. So, too, had Gordon been drinking and he was only thirteen-years-old. Although no one ever knew where the young people got the booze, it was common knowledge that it was readily available and there were those who would supply it. Things haven't changed much other than the legal age being lowered from twenty-one to eighteen. Now that's a real step forward for society! The truck belonged to Gordon's dad and we learned later that Gordon had insisted on driving home and Bill had permitted it. It was not unusual for young people (boys) to be driving on the country roads as they helped out on the family farm. They often learned to drive as early as eleven or twelve-years-of age. Bill was thrown out of the truck and killed as the truck rolled on top of him. The policeman who attended the accident said he died instantly. I wonder if they say that to be kind to families. Gordon was also ejected but thrown clear. He was critically injured and yet still managed to crawl the half-mile to their home to get help. Gordon spent many months in hospital recuperating and still bears the scars of that fateful day.

The next few days passed in a blur. Neighbors came and went. "If there's anything we can do? How can we help?" But, what could they do? Everyone wanted to help. "Leave us alone!!" My head screamed but my mouth was silent. "I know just how you feel," declared one of the neighbors. "Like hell you do," I wanted to scream, but my mouth wouldn't work. How could anyone possibly know how I felt? I just wanted to run away and escape the madness, the insanity that had taken over our house.

The funeral came and went and I only remember the rain. It was so fitting. The rain simply blended with the tears streaming down my face. This was one of those times when I felt alone in a crowd. I don't know who was there and who wasn't. It didn't matter. I just wanted to be alone. It's funny, there were many times in my life when I felt alone in a crowd and the loneliness threatened to engulf me. There were times when I felt invisible and so alone in that crowded household that we called home. Today, when all I wanted was to be alone, I felt as though my space was being invaded and I hardly had room to breathe. It was so crowded I was sure my very thoughts were bouncing into the brains of others. Hmm! I wonder if that's where the term "brain drain" originated. Just a thought!

A few days later I returned to school. Everything felt so different. Certainly, things had changed in our household. It was a strange phenomenon in which this person who no longer existed controlled our every thought and our every action. He was there but he wasn't. We couldn't speak his name. We couldn't play his music and we couldn't grieve openly. It seemed Mom could not bear to have anything around that reminded her of Bill.

And since we couldn't acknowledge his death, therefore it just didn't happen. Was it possible that Bill had never really existed and had never been a part of our family? Maybe it was all just a bad dream. But if it was a bad dream, it affected everyone and somehow we were all part of the same nightmare. At times I wondered if perhaps Bill was the only one who really mattered and was truly loved. There were, after all, nine other children needing a hug and needing to hear they were loved and that there was room for them in the hearts of our parents. But outwardly we were not a demonstrative family. Some things were just understood. I only understood the pain as our family became more dysfunctional. We, as siblings, became caregivers for each other. We didn't talk of Bill. It was as though he had never been. And yet his life and death were forever a part of who we were. Bill's death changed our household in ways too numerous to count. Mom became chronically ill. Today she would probably have been diagnosed as suffering from depression. She spent much of each day in bed and it seemed as though she was always sick. I remember thinking she was a hypochondriac. I resented missing school and having to stay home to cook, clean and look after my siblings. After all, they were not my kids. My parents chose to have twelve children. I shouldn't have to suffer for their decisions.

"Mom, have you never heard of birth control?" I asked on learning that Mom was pregnant again. I felt embarrassed by her pregnancy and the response to my question was a sound slap across the face. That was probably the only time my mother slapped me across the face but I can still feel the sting and at that moment my determination to leave home increased to an all time high. I so resented having to take on what I believed to be responsibilities that should never have been mine.

I hated missing school since that was my ticket to freedom. It was my temporary escape from reality. I could hide there. I could dream of what it would be like to be somebody. I could read stories and transport myself to fabulous, exotic places far away. School was my safety net. I was good at school and could feel good about myself. I wasn't popular on the playground. I wasn't good at sports; but I could spell; I could do reading, writing and arithmetic. I excelled at spelling bees and math quizzes. Actually I do remember my dad being proud of me and expecting me to do well. My dad was a very proud man. He was proud of the Whitfield name (although I don't exactly know why.) Even though we were poor, he was too proud to take a handout and always said you didn't buy on credit. If you couldn't afford it you didn't buy it. I remember in Saskatchewan when the government brought in the family allowance. My dad was indignant and even though the checks came in Mom's name Dad declared, "We'll accept no welfare in this household," and promptly returned the checks. Eventually they were accepted but my dad's pride remained strong.

I'm grateful for a couple of dear friends in whom I could at least confide the loss, the sadness and the grief around my brother's death. Of course, I couldn't tell the secret things that had gone on behind closed doors. I couldn't air our dirty laundry in public. But I could grieve and I could cry in the safety of my friends' homes. My mom's younger sister was always there for me. I would walk the two miles north to their home simply just to talk to her. She was frequently at our home. She and Mom were close as sisters and friends who supported one another in joy and sorrow. They helped each other endure the many hardships of the times.

Part of me felt so sad. I had not experienced the death of anyone close to me before. It was as though my heart was being ripped out of my chest. At times I cried as though the tears would never stop and I was sure I was going to throw-up. I couldn't eat and couldn't stand the pity from all the neighbors. And I felt so guilty. I had killed my brother.

For what seemed like years I had prayed for my brother to die. I had dreamt about all the ways that might happen. Over and over in my mind I pictured this moment. Perhaps he'd die of that heart problem they'd been concerned about when he had rheumatic fever; perhaps a train'd hit him; perhaps he'd die in a car accident. It was my only hope for escape—escape from the madness, the abuse, the degradation and the shame. And so I prayed; and then it happened. I killed him. God had heard my prayer and answered it. "But no God, this cannot be happening. I didn't mean it, honest I didn't." The guilt increased tenfold. Not only was I dirty, I was also a murderer. My brother was dead and I was to blame. I think I always believed God answered prayer but this was too much. The loving God of my childhood, in whose presence I felt warm and protected, seemed distant and I wondered if I had even become invisible to God. I was so confused. If God heard and answered my prayer then I couldn't be invisible. Perhaps I just wished I was and in that way could hide even from God. I became afraid to talk to God. What if I prayed or thought something horrible and it happened again.

I don't recall exactly when it started—or even when I realized it was wrong, but I remember the secrecy, the feelings of being dirty and full of shame. "I'm going to tell Mom." I declared over and over again. The response was laughter and ridicule. "Who'd believe you? You're only a child." And quickly I was silenced. He was right, of course.

But how could no one have known? Or did they just turn a blind eye to the incest? Was it just part of the insanity, of the dysfunction? My two older brothers shared the bedroom at the top of the stairs on the right. Mom and Dad's bedroom was at the top of the stairs to the left. Our house was not huge and there were many of us crowded into that small space. I lived in fear of discovery and hope of someone finding out and putting a stop to the pain.

Yes, I was indeed the invisible child and my brother could do what he wished. He was right. No one would believe me. He was the adored, eldest son who could do no wrong. I too, adored him, in my own way. I adored him and hated him. My dad was an alcoholic and Bill followed in his footsteps. On weekends he and his friends would go out drinking and dancing. The next morning the repeated refrain was that he didn't remember what he had done the night before. I knew he and his friends were scrappers and went looking for fights. I hated that. I didn't believe he couldn't remember. I believe he didn't want to remember what he had done. Perhaps, a little like me, he experienced shame—but probably not. My brother was so handsome and so worldly. He had lots of friends and was very popular. I became his willing accomplice. I didn't resist his attention—he loved me. I was his kid sister. Even when his bidding became sexual, I just obeyed and later wondered why I didn't just say "no." I don't remember all the details but I have vivid memories of being in his bed, being fondled and touched all over.

As I began to approach the teenage years I felt sick at what we were doing and I begged to stop this insanity. But my pleas went unheeded and he began to threaten me. He would tell Mom if I didn't co-operate.

Bill was the firstborn child and that was as it should be. A boy first—he was my parent's dream child. He was a rather serious, good-looking, smart child from whom much was expected. At age thirteen, (which would make me about eight-years-old) he had developed rheumatic fever, and was very sick. There were concerns about the effects on his heart in later years. The most significant thing I remember about rheumatic fever was that the soles of his feet turned black and he was unable to walk. He was hospitalized for a long time and then bedridden when he came home. Bill recovered but he never went back to school. He quit school to stay home and help on the farm. That was not unusual at that time in history. A high-school education was not seen to be a necessity and many young men quit school to farm with their fathers. Bill, with Dad's help, eventually bought my Grandpa's land, south of our farm, and Dad and Bill set up farming together.

I adored my oldest brother and as he began to go out in the evenings with his friends, I took great pride in being asked to polish his shoes or press his shirt or slacks. Shoes netted me ten cents, while shirts and slacks were worth twenty-five cents. It took me an hour of babysitting to earn that much. Perhaps my financial good fortune was payment for my silence. In any event that seemed like a lot of money to me at the time and I didn't turn it down.

And so I carried my own memories with no outlet for my feelings and no one to talk to. I didn't dare talk, Bill was dead and so I would have to live with my own dirty secrets and the guilt of having been responsible for his death. I believed God answered prayer but this was too much. The loving God of my childhood, in whose presence I felt warm and protected, seemed distant and I wondered if I had even become invisible to God. Yet I knew that God heard my prayers. Hadn't God answered that horrible prayer I had prayed so many times? I became afraid to talk to God. What if I prayed or thought something horrible and it happened again?

I guarded my thoughts and tried hard to bury the guilt but it persisted and refused to let go of me. I never talked of my experiences. I couldn't. I had killed my brother and felt so condemned and guilty. I desperately tried to put it out of my mind and sometimes was more successful than others.

Mom and Dad drifted further apart and seemed to simply live in the same household. (Yet, two more children were conceived and brought into this world after Bill died.) My oldest sister had married and she and Mom were pregnant at the same time. How disgusting!! I was sixteen-years-old and felt I should have been enjoying life and going out with my friends. Fat chance there was of that happening! My boyfriend wanted us to run away and elope. He was nineteen and I was sixteen. My dad didn't approve of him. Dad said he was too old for me. The idea of running off to elope seemed romantic and enticing. Something inside me knew that I had to graduate from high school and the only way that was going to happen was for me to stay in school and that meant staying on the farm. I had to escape the poverty but first I had to get an education in order to do that.

The fights and the yelling on the home front became more frequent and I dreaded returning each evening to our family farm. Dad had been a binge alcoholic for many years and his anger seemed to increase and threaten to explode with no place to go. Any happiness I'd experienced as a child disappeared. Things went from bad to worse. Murphy's law kicked in big time. As Dad's temper flared, my next oldest brother took the brunt of that anger. Oh, for sure he was a troubled child. Dick had been with Bill and Gordon the night of the accident. He had just been dropped off and was not yet asleep when we received the news of the accident. Dick had worshipped the ground Bill walked on and tried to emulate him. I remember the nightmares, not mine—Dick's, the waking up in the night screaming with terror and being yelled at to shut up and go back to sleep. Eventually, Dick just left home.

Dick and I were good friends as well as siblings. Dick was only one-and-one half years older than me and we spent healthy time together. Unlike me, Dick hated school and when he left home he became a jockey and rode racehorses. I let my imagination run wild and glamorized the life he led. My disdain for my dad grew ten-fold after Dick left home. At times I hated my dad, almost as much as I hated myself. I missed Dick terribly and looked forward to receiving his infrequent letters. He was my best friend. I once received a note scribbled on about three feet of toilet paper written from a truck stop along his travels. That was more indicative than my wild imagination of how he survived in the world of hard knocks. But this is Dick's story and so I only include what I need to in order to tell my own story.

I was not a very happy youngster and looked towards the day when I could finally leave home. It's natural for young people to look with anticipation to the time when they grow up and leave home to make their own way in the world. I longed for that day, probably more than most. This longing absorbed my every waking hour and created in me a drivenness; a need to prove myself and to succeed. The scriptures keep proving themselves over and over again to me. I have discovered that God can use all things for good. As a young teenager I swore I would never let anything control my mind and vowed never to drink. I have kept that vow although it has moved from being an angry vow to being a lifelong choice as part of who I am.

Still, my teenage years had some highlights and things were not all doom and gloom. Much to my surprise, I survived growing up a poor "Whitfield brat." I worked hard at school and can remember waiting until everyone else was in bed, then sitting at the kitchen table doing homework by the light of a coal oil lantern. We didn't have electricity in our house back then. The dedication to learning paid off. I remember waiting in anticipation for the mail to come containing my transcript of senior matriculation departmental exams. These were sent out by the government and didn't arrive until late in the summer. When that day finally came, I stood holding the envelope for a long time as though the marks would reveal themselves without me having to actually open the envelope. It took all the courage I could muster and then a sigh of relief. I had graduated with a complete grade twelve. I was elated.

I had aspirations of becoming a schoolteacher. I had spent some time during my grade twelve year as a substitute teacher which was a privilege given to those expressing a desire to attend university or Teacher's college after completing high school. We had been encouraged to submit our applications as well so that upon receipt of our transcript of marks

we could gain immediate admission. I had applied and was accepted at the University of
Saskatchewan for the fall term to begin studying for a degree in education. I never told
anyone of having received either the acceptance or of having responded. "No, I would not be
attending the fall session." I knew there was no money for me to go to University.

After graduation I applied for and got a job in a general store selling everything from
food to high fashion apparel. I remember feeling good about myself as I was asked in the job
interview why they should hire me. "Because you need a clerk, and I need a job." I replied
and was hired on the spot. Dad was so proud of me. Achievements and status were
important to Dad. I recalled other times in my life when I knew that Dad was proud of me. I
was always an "A" student and Dad bragged about that. He drove me to public speaking
competitions and made sure everyone knew I was his daughter. The joy in these times were
often overshadowed when the drunkenness kicked in and seemed to loom larger than life
itself.

Yet, in many ways, Dad tried so hard. As I began my new job and entered the world
of independence I began to make the break from all that was in my past. I returned to that
farm every weekend until I got married. Dad, faithfully, came to pick me up after work
every Saturday night and then drove me back to work every Monday night. Sundays and
Mondays were my days off. I enjoyed those drives, when we didn't stop at the pub, and
actually began to develop a relationship of respect and gain an understanding of who my dad
was as I learned of some of the struggles on his journey. I didn't pay much attention but
realize now that Dad gave up his Saturday night for me. That was pub night wasn't it? I
wonder what that was like for him.

Those times with my dad became treasured memories. I discovered that I didn't really hate my dad. I hated that he drank and the effects it had on our family as a whole. Perhaps I had to leave home to see the bigger picture. It wasn't much but it was a beginning. Beginnings beg continuance and the resulting journey can bring healing and forgiveness.

Memories

The overcast skies reflected my spirit as I knelt at the graveside. Tears flowed as the years rolled back. I was transported back in time to the year 1969. The date was June 7th. It was late Saturday afternoon. A couple of hours earlier I had bid farewell to my husband. "See ya later, Boss," were his parting words to me. "Boss" was his pet name for me, an inside joke between the two of us. Those were the last words I would ever hear him say.

My thoughts were jumbled, the memories somewhat confused in my mind. I don't recall who made that horrible phone call but the message and the instructions were clear. Lovall, my husband of six and one-half short years, had been in a car accident and was en route by ambulance to Thompson General Hospital, "Meet us at the hospital," the voice said. "We'll be there in ten minutes."

Carrol and Garry, Lovall's sister and her husband appeared, as though out of nowhere, to drive me to the hospital. I was grateful they didn't want me to go alone. On arrival we were escorted to a cordoned off semi-private area of emergency. A terror had gripped my heart; I shivered and suddenly felt a horrible chill. An ominous cloud had settled in. I was so cold. I didn't want to see him, but I had to. His badly broken unconscious body was swathed in bandages. His face was all that was completely exposed. The face of the man I loved, and had loved since childhood, was so deathly white. But No! I would not allow my mind to go there.

"There's not much hope." Dr. Spooner spoke in a monotone voice. "We cannot get a blood pressure reading." I was numb. I stood by the bedside of my dying husband and prayed that it would not be so. Please God don't let him die! Perhaps God had deaf ears that day, or perhaps he was too busy to head my prayers. I only know they were not answered.

Lovall "expired" at 7:15 on the evening of June 7th, 1969, according to the newspaper report. He never regained consciousness. I hate that word "expired." Why couldn't they just outright say he'd died? A part of me died with him that night.

We returned from the hospital to the sound of the telephone ringing. Lovall and I had watched this home being built and planned to live here into old age. The phone interrupted my thoughts. It was Sternie, Lovall's brother. "How is Lovall?" he asked. Intuitively he sensed something was dreadfully wrong and that Lovall had been in an accident. I've heard that happens sometimes with twins and that a special bond between them is strong enough for them to sense when something is wrong. Although Sternie and Lovall were not twins, with Lovall being eleven months older than Sternie, they were as close as any two brothers could be. I sobbed out the news that Lovall had not survived the accident and we cried together. Sternie was a quadriplegic having suffered a broken neck and numerous other injuries from a car accident when he was eighteen. And now Lovall was dead.

People came to offer condolences and make small talk. "Can we help? What can we do?" I don't know. What's to do? The June rains fell in harmony with my inner self, at times falling softly, so sadly and at other times lashing out with a harshness that cried as though in agreement with my bitterness and anger. How could this be happening? "Why me Lord?" It was all so unfair.

In a daze and with much help from family and friends I went through the motions of arranging a funeral and wrapping up the details of a lifetime. We had been married six and a half short years and had two beautiful children. Our lives had seemed nearly perfect- perhaps too perfect. Oh, God – life is so cruel. How does one tie up loose ends and continue on as only half a person? "For this cause a man shall leave his father and his mother, and shall cleave to his wife; and they shall become one flesh." (Genesis 2:24) I felt as though part of my flesh was literally been ripped to shreds. Lovall and I had been as one flesh. We completed each other. Was it possible for me to continue without him? I wasn't even sure I wanted to.

I was paralyzed. I tried to block out the details of that horrible accident and then the picture appeared on the front page of *The Thompson Citizen* daily news. I didn't tell them they could print that picture. *This is my life, not yours.* The stark reality of life – the more sensational, the more horrific- that's the stuff that sells papers. People don't matter. Feelings just tend to get in the road and then get trod on.

Oh, yes, the funeral, it needed to be taken care of. Meet with the minister – try to put on a brave face, or at least be coherent. All this was new to me. I wasn't sure what needed to be done. Pallbearers would be needed to carry my beloved husband's body to its final resting place. But there would be no resting place for me. I'd never been to a funeral here in Thompson. In fact I've not even been out to the cemetery. I think it's north of town. I guessed I'd find out soon enough. Sometimes people are taken home to their birthplace to be buried, but this place had been our home and so it seemed this was the appropriate place for

Lovall's burial. Um, pallbearers, yes, perhaps Ted, Dave and Jim would do that. At that moment I didn't know who else to ask and I thought I needed six of them. Those three were his closest friends. My mind wandered to the power toboggan club, the races; the hours spent modifying engines for peak performance at races and the fun times shared with our friends. There'd be no more of those.

Somehow the details got taken care of and the day of the funeral came and went. In the days leading up to that final farewell, I remember contacting people. My parents and my Uncle Sid left Saskatchewan immediately to make the trek to Thompson. Lovall's family came as well. Lovall's mom had died of cancer just six months earlier.

I really didn't want so many people around but that's how funerals are. Some good friends took care of Starla and Sternie (my daughter and son) to allow me time and space to make arrangements. The United Church had become a big part of my life and our minister was so helpful. The day of the funeral poured rain and as my parents supported me from the church to the graveside the rain on my cheeks felt right as it mixed with my tears and created the appropriate atmosphere for the hardest day of my life.

"Keep a stiff upper lip," my Grandpa used to say, "You're made of good stuff." I didn't always feel that but there was a side of me that needed to portray strength to the outside world. Perhaps that's what Grandpa meant.

One of the managers at INCO, where Lovall had worked as welder and mechanic, had become friends with us and now pulled some strings for me to get admission to Keewatin Community College in The Pas, Manitoba. The Pas is 143 miles south of Thompson and offers a variety of adult education programs along with University Transfer courses. I had previously taken a couple of distance education transfer courses and the possibility of entering the world of study appealed to me. And so, within a couple of months I headed back to school. It was all so overwhelming and perhaps it was happening too soon. Before I knew it I was thrust into the school environment, studying, doing homework and writing exams, as well as being a mom to two now fatherless children. It was tough.

Through it all, I was yanked back and forth like a puppet on a string; from the present, to memories of the past and then jerked forward to focusing on the future and what needed to be done. It was so damned hard. I didn't want to do this anymore.

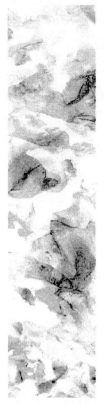

My Mind

My mind's a mess, it's all screwed up,
and why I do not know.
My thoughts, they race and
sleep won't come.
No rest for my weary soul.

I've travelled far and I've travelled wide.
I've seen so many things.
But peace won't come though
the sun has set
and the darkness of evening springs.

My aimless mind just wanders on;
it's darting here and there.
As I gaze out of the window,
it's closing in (the world) with a
quickness I cannot bear.

Freedom escapes me, life's taken its toll.
Freedom I long for and yet with
it comes certain fear.
Fear of the unknown, of what lies ahead.
Out there, beyond the years — my mind
plays tricks.

The river's high. The bridge is too.
God, please forgive me now,
But life's too hard to go on living.
I must escape the pain.

The pain of what I do not know
and yet I must.
I speed on down the highway,
what if, what if,
If just perhaps I turn the wheel — escape
will then be mine.
A split second is all it'll take. Goodbye
cruel world, goodbye.

Screeeech! Crash!!! (Darkness)

(A *Family Affair- jorie's story* 17)

At fourteen years of age I walked into the kitchen of our old farmhouse and

announced boldly, "Mom, today I met the man I'm going to marry."

"Puppy love," declared my mom.

July 12^{th,} 1959, my older sister and I had plans to attend the Saskatoon Exhibition and so I was permitted to spend the night with her in her apartment in town. She worked late that night and we had to catch the early morning train. It would pull out at 4:30 a.m. "I don't feel like sleeping. Let's go for a coke." She didn't have to convince me. We headed off to the Town and Country Café. It was the local teenage hangout—complete with jukebox and a space to jive at the back of the restaurant. We weren't there long when in walked my sister's boy friend with a group of his friends. Soon they came and joined us, that is, all except Lovall. "Oh, he's shy," they said. Something in his shyness caught my attention and our eyes locked. That shy young man in the turquoise shirt is a picture engraved on the canvass of my memory.

Five years later we were married in the United Church in my hometown of Biggar, Saskatchewan. Our small family reception was held in the Banquet Room of the Town and Country Café where we first met. We lived for a short while in Melville, Saskatchewan before moving to the northern mining community of Thompson, Manitoba. Thompson was experiencing a boom and there was an excitement in being part of the formation of a new town. Everyone had come from somewhere else to seek the promised fortunes of the North. North-of- 55 t-shirts and paraphernalia were common gifts taken home for family and friends. There was a sense of pride in being part of new frontiers. We were truly sixties pioneers. Meeting people was easy and we were soon involved with the snowmobile club and the bowling league. There were many newly-weds, like Lovall and myself, and young families who got together often for fellowship and competition. It certainly was a young people's town. On those rare occasions when you saw any elderly people, you knew they were visiting.

The job market in Thompson and the good money to be made there enticed people from all over to brave the cold winters, and the black flies and mosquitoes in the summer, to make Thompson home. Shortly after we established our home there, it became a temporary home for numerous family members and friends as they too decided Thompson was the place to be.

Life wasn't all easy, but it was good. We worked hard and played hard. Lovall worked for the International Nickel Company (INCO). In many ways Thompson was a company town. As the town grew so, of course, did the services that were offered there. I worked for the Hudson's Bay store, before my kid's, between my kids and after my kid's. The thought of being a stay-at-home mom was never part of the plan. Lovall dreamed of having his own business and the two of us worked hard towards fulfilling that dream. As the dream became a reality we knew that it would take time and we would continue to work elsewhere as we developed the business. In our spare time, I looked after the bookkeeping details while Lovall sold, repaired and serviced small engines and snowmobiles. He had just gotten the Chrysler boat and motor franchise and was excited about the future possibilities of becoming an independent entrepreneur. The architectural plans were complete and the location for development had been approved. Arrangements for financing were in the works and we were awaiting final approval from our bank.

Lovall headed off to Winnipeg to pick up his first shipment of boats and motors. He had recently purchased a new Ford pickup and today was taking two of our neighbors with him to help with loading our shipment. Winnipeg was an eight-hour drive, 600 miles south of Thompson. Highway 391 had improved considerably from when we arrived there in 1963. We had traveled to Thompson by train, as the road at that time was what they called a winter road. The road was only partially paved and not passable in the summer. Within a couple of years most of the road was paved. There was still a stretch that was gravel and dust hung heavy in the air. Visibility was always poor. There is a place called SOAB creek about 40 miles or so south of Thompson. Rumor says SOAB stands for "Son-of-a-bitch" of a place. The name still stands today.

Lovall collided head on with a gravel truck. He never saw it coming. The trucker escaped injury while Lovall's passengers were taken to Thompson Hospital, treated for minor injuries and released. Lovall "expired" at 7:15 that evening. And my life changed forever.

My children were five and one when their dad died. Some well meaning friends advised against the children attending the funeral. It wasn't necessary for them to be immersed in such grief. And so they were whisked off to the neighbors for the duration. But I needed them and they needed me. It was our loss. As if we could protect them from grief! They'd just lost their dad.

Years later there was a sense of sadness around knowing that I was not present for my kids in their grief and for that I am deeply sorry. And so I embark on another journey. I gather together pictures and mementos as I begin to piece together the fragments of Lovall's life. I have this need to share it with my children, to share who he was as a person, how special he was and how very much he loved them, how much he loved all of us.

Initially, my intentions were that this memory book would be completed for my children. As the project took shape it grew in scope and Lovall's family, especially his brother Sternie, for whom our son was named, and his sister Carrol, who was Lovall's baby sister and had lived with us for a period of time after she graduated from high-school, became recipients as well. As the book unfolded there was the realization that I was doing it not only for them, but also for myself. It was part of my own latent grief work.

Sternie, my oldest son, sat at my kitchen table and the tears streamed down his cheeks as he read the memory book. Tears dripped off his mustache and beard, which he sported proudly declaring his masculinity. My heart ached, my tears joined his and I offered a hug to my grown up son. There were no words – simply a release of pent up anger and grief. Grief he had buried deep inside for so long with no place to go. It has been well hidden. The anger has not been so easily hidden. My heart broke and I was torn up inside as I watched my son express feelings hidden for so many years. He's always been a loner and has carried everything inside, all bottled up. At times his anger and frustration has found strange and sometimes harmful ways of finding expression over the years. But that's his story and I won't encroach other than to say that there was a chink in the dam that day and as it began to let go my son cried unashamedly and for that moment his anger subsided. We talked for hours that day. We shared our tears, our grief, our memories and our love and for that moment that was enough. The healing could begin.

Honor Thy Father and Thy Mother

On August 14th, 2005, I congregated with others from my past as we gathered in community at the Leney Cemetery to remember loved ones buried here. Some of the faces were familiar while others were faces of those I didn't know and yet they recognized me as one of the Whitfield girls. I could hear my father's voice saying, "Oh, you must remember so and so. They farm just down the correction line," or "They're from Perdue," or "They live just out of Biggar." Dad knew everyone and expected that we did as well.

The freshly cut grass and manicured gravesites bore evidence to the many hours of labor put in as preparation for this night. One might say it was a labor of love, a way of honoring those who had gone before. The Leney Cemetery committee takes great pride in maintaining the grounds and hosting this yearly memorial service. Volunteers do all the maintenance and upkeep. Dad served on that committee for many years and took pride in knowing it was one of the best-kept cemeteries in the country. When he died he left a sizeable amount to Leney Cemetery to ensure continued care.

The Service began. We prayed, listened to a scripture passage from Isaiah and sang an old familiar hymn. It seemed fitting as we remembered those who had passed from this world to the next. Those who had died in the past year were named aloud and the minister paused after each name. This year there were only nine names but subconsciously I heard the names of my parents, Ronald and Laura Whitfield, in that list as it was read aloud. I could picture Dad wandering among the headstones, taking time to stop and read each one. He would recognize the names of those buried here.

My father was intrigued with cemeteries. In 1989 I accompanied my parents on a trip to New Zealand. Almost before we were unpacked and settled in our hotel, Dad spotted a cemetery and we toured it looking for familiar names. My dad's Uncle Clem immigrated to New Zealand at the time my grandfather came to Canada. We went to New Zealand with the express purpose of connecting with the Whitfield relatives. It was the trip of a lifetime. (Except for the cemetery tours.) I never quite understood my dad's fascination with cemeteries. I just accepted it as a quirky part of who he was. Tonight, before the service began, I found myself wandering among the grave sites, reading the names and conjuring up memories of those I knew and pondering on the lives of the many strangers laid to rest in the confines of this remote cemetery. (The apple really doesn't fall far from the apple tree.)

My parents are both buried here. Dad died three years ago and Mom seven years prior. Their ashes are interred in the same plot in which my brother's body was buried back in 1959. Roses and a straw bale adorned with wheat and cattails have been lovingly placed on the graves by two of my sisters and myself. Mom loved the roses, while Dad was a farmer through and through. We laugh as we reminisce and we shed a few tears. We come face-to-face with our own mortality and the reality of the fragility of life. These, our parents and our grandparents, were real living, breathing, people just a few short years ago and their lives mattered. They are part of who we are. My grandparents' final resting place is next door (so to speak) and so tonight I remember them all.

This has become an annual pilgrimage for many of our family, but tonight is different somehow. The memories of my parents are especially poignant and there is a strange reality that enfolds me in the intensity of missing them. It would be great to hear their voices one more time, perhaps even to be able to say "I love you," once again.

As scripture passages are read from Matthew's gospel and the first Epistle of John, the Beatitudes again assure us of God's comfort in times of mourning as do John's words. My mind wanders to another scripture verse, one that speaks specifically to why I am here tonight.

"Honor thy father and thy mother, as the LORD thy God hath commanded thee; that thy days may be prolonged, and that it may go well with you…"
(Deuteronomy 5:16)

We didn't go to church, but we certainly heard the Ten Commandments. This commandment was, at times, particularly difficult to obey. What did it mean to honor my parents and did I really have to honor my father when he came stumbling home, stinking rotten drunk?

Memories of other times and other places come flooding back. I find myself in the University Hospital.

"Margie, you know I find it difficult to sleep. I wonder if you would come up later tonight and sit with me a while? A cup of coffee would be nice." Mom spoke from the confines of her hospital bed. Margie was a term of endearment restricted for use by my mom, my aunts and my granny.

"Sure Mom. I'll be back shortly." I replied. Mom liked her coffee strong and up straight. The coffee from the cafeteria at this time of night should fit that bill.

Visiting time was over and Dad was about to retire for the night to the Outpatient Residence often referred to simply as the OPR. The OPR provided special, inexpensive, accommodations for families of those suffering from cancer or other terminal illnesses. The doors locked at eleven o'clock at night and Dad was exhausted and ready for a good night's sleep. Mom had earlier been diagnosed with bowel cancer and was a patient at the University Hospital where I was one of the staff chaplains. The cancer specialist at the Cross Cancer Institute had called us for a family conference and demonstrated through diagrams the extent of Mom's cancer. "There is nothing we can do. The cancer has wrapped itself around all the vital organs. Surgery is out of the question. We will make you as comfortable as possible and try to control the pain," she said. Mom had already been through the gamut of surgery, radiation and chemotherapy. She had made up her mind that she would not undergo any further treatment and so the Doctor's announcement merely confirmed her own decision. She would wait in the University Hospital until a bed became available in Palliative Care at Red Deer Regional Hospital.

Dad and I walked in silence to the entrance of OPR and paused at the doorway.

"Goodnight Dad. See you in the morning. Breakfast at 7:00?"

"Great. See you then. Goodnight dear."

As I turned to go for the coffee Mom had requested, I thanked God for the privilege afforded me as staff chaplain. I was not restricted to visiting hours and had the freedom to come and go as I pleased. One-on-one time with Mom was precious. It had been a rare commodity in my life and so I relished this time. I returned to Mom's room to the pleasant discovery that she had fallen asleep. I pulled a chair close to the bed and just sat quietly contemplating the future. Mom was dying. What would it be like without her? I wondered and allowed my mind to wander.

I never really knew my mom. She was a private person in many ways and throughout my childhood and teenage years, I never felt close to her. There were moments when I felt her love, moments when she'd go out of her way to make things special for me. One night she stayed up all night making me a new pink and black blouse to wear to a school dance. I was a big Elvis fan at the time and pink and black were his colors. The blouse was truly a thing of beauty and I wore it with pride. Mom was a great seamstress and with a magical touch old garments became new creations that rivaled anything you would buy in either the Hudson's Bay or Eaton's. I think my mom was the originator of the recycling concept. She did it so well.

My parents were a strange mix. They came from very different backgrounds, which was not readily acceptable in those times. Mom was French and Dad was English. We used to joke that the war between the French and the English had never really ended. It just moved to our house. Mom was brought up in a strict Roman Catholic home while Dad came from an Anglican background. "High Anglican", my granny declared which really was what in England was called The Church of England. Regardless, I didn't know my father's folks to be much for churchgoing and so perhaps it was easier for Dad to move away from his faith background than it was for Mom. My dad smoked and drank and Mom did neither of those things.

I've heard it said, "Change is the only constant," and our lives seemed to bear out the truth of that statement. Change in itself is neither good nor bad but the changes wrought by the circumstances of life can have positive or negative effects. Bringing together two such diverse personalities, as Mom and Dad, in the holy estate of matrimony solicits change of magnanimous proportion. To my dad it was, "All just part of the hand we are dealt."

After the death of my brother, Mom, on the advice of her doctor, started smoking. It would calm her nerves, he said. (Wow! How things have changed!) Eventually my dad gave up smoking and drinking, but neither of those things happened while I lived at home.

Strange mixture or not, my parents survived fifty-seven years of marriage before my mom died of cancer. I'm not sure what brought them together in the first place and Mom and Dad weren't much for sharing their stories with us, but Grandpa was a great storyteller. Problem was, the twinkle in his eye led one to wonder how much of the story was true and how much was fabricated to delight us children. Mom and Dad were too busy raising all of us and surviving the day-to-day grind to bother much with story telling.

I've probably learned more about my parents' courtship days and their decision to marry from Auntie Marion and Auntie Jean than either of my parents would have liked me to know. Auntie Marion laughs as she recalls, "Your mom declared, 'If you won't let us get married, I'll just get pregnant and then we'll have to get married,' and I think she meant it." Back in those days a pregnancy almost always meant a forced wedding. Apparently Mom knew how to get her own way. I wonder if she actually would have carried out that threat.

Auntie Marion remembers my dad as "that handsome blond Englishman from the North," and delights in telling of seeing him ride over the hills on horseback to come courting my mom.

My parents had a love for music and were probably the best dancers on any dance floor. I learned to dance on my father's feet. I would stand on his feet and he would whirl off to the popular big band music. Dad could keep time but couldn't sing a note (a trait I inherited from him). Mom was the musician in our family. She could sing and play guitar. Auntie Jean has talked to us about how she and Mom were part of a musical band in their teen years. I've seen enough pictures of them that I can imagine them making merriment and just having a ball. Mom would gather us around, play guitar and lead a sing-along in the early days. It was great fun.

I finished my coffee, gave Mom a kiss on the cheek, being careful not to awaken her, and walked quietly out, down the hallway, to the sleep-room that I had laid claim to for now.

Each night I would accompany Dad to the OPR, pick up a coffee and return to Mom's room. If Mom were asleep I would sit for a couple of hours, hold her hand and simply remember. My memories supplied a private Technicolor home mini-movie. Tonight's scene opens in the kitchen of our old farmhouse.

"You'll do as I say," yelled Mom. "You're not going, and that's that." The smack across my face with the spatula she had in her hand echoed loudly. It stung me too. Perhaps the shock hurt more than the act itself. Mom rarely ever laid a hand on her daughters. She yelled lots, but not usually at me. Perhaps that's because, to a great extent I was the good kid. I tried hard to do what was expected of me. I was a pleaser and hated confrontation. I was a timid child in many ways, having learned early in life that I, and all children, were to be seen and not heard. But I was no longer a child. I was sixteen and old enough to be left responsible for looking after my younger brothers and sisters. This was not fair.

"But Mom, you promised. This party has been planned for weeks. It's our last get together before the school year ends," I said between sobs.

"I don't care. We have company and you're not going!" Weeks ago students from our high school had planned this year-end bonfire and wiener roast on a neighboring farm. Mom knew about it and had given me permission to go. But now, the night of the party, we had company and so Mom had changed her mind.

Hurt and angry, I retreated to my room. "How could she treat me like a kid and yell like a banshee in front of everyone? How embarrassing is that?" I muttered as I stormed off to my room, slamming the door behind me. "I'll just stay in my room all evening. If only I were more like Dick. I'd have the guts to just go." But I couldn't do that. I was not Dick. I was Marj, and so tonight I would escape to my own private world. I would get lost in the fantasy of a book and transport myself off on an exotic journey somewhere far from here.

This particular mini-home movie was brief, but it opened the floodgates for other memories and for a couple of hours my mind wandered freely with no set path. I wondered about my mom's childhood. What was life like for her? My grandmother had outlived three husbands, which meant my mom had two step-dads. What was that like? As a single mom, Granny spent a number of years cleaning houses for other people to earn enough to support herself and her two daughters. Life must have been hard. I envisioned Mom and Auntie Jean as little girls. Who looked after them while Granny was off cleaning houses?

Finally, my imagination quieted and my mind settled down. I was tired. It was after 2:00 am. I had to work early in the morning. I leaned over, kissed Mom gently and slipped out of the room.

Other nights, when Mom was wide-awake we would talk.

"Mom, did you and Dad really plan on having twelve kids? What was it like raising all of us? You used to say things like, 'They're cheaper by the dozen,' and 'there's always room for one more.' Sometimes there was hardly room for all of us." Mom simply laughed in response and changed the subject. But my questions did not cease.

"Mom, I know you left your church. What was it like turning your back on God and your faith? Didn't you miss going to church? Where is God in your life? Did you really want to be a nun? I used to admire Auntie Madeline and I dreamt of becoming a nun. Did you know that mum?

"Well, yes, it was difficult, but you know dear, faith is in your heart. It doesn't have to be spoken. I discovered I didn't need to go to church to believe in God. He's always in my heart. I know He's with me. My faith is still strong. I couldn't have survived without my faith. But I was not really meant to be a nun. I actually left the novitiate long before I knew your father. I just was not cut out for that life. I love children and yes, we always wanted a big family. The religious training was good training though and gave me a foundation for my faith."

I had never heard Mom talk about God or her beliefs. She, like Mary, pondered these things and kept them in her heart. We prayed together that night as mother and daughter for the very first time.

"Mom, I really don't know that much about your life. What dreams did you hold in your heart as a young woman? Did you give them all up for us? What was important in your life? Was I important? Did I matter in the big scheme of things? Did you really love me?"

"Oh, yes dear, I love you and always have. But Margie, dear, you were the strong one. I always knew you'd be okay. I didn't have to worry about you. You were always so independent. You could always manage on your own. Sometimes it seemed you didn't need us."

"I wished you had told me that. I thought you didn't care. I often thought it would be better around home if I weren't there. Why didn't you ever say, I love you."

We talked long into the night. We spoke those three precious words rarely heard in our household. "I love you!" We cried as we held each other and the tears were good tears.

Mom spent two precious weeks at the University Hospital and then lived out the final six months of her life in palliative care at Red Deer Regional Hospital. God looked out and saw me with an aching heart, needing a mother's love and gave that special gift of conversation, prayer, time and healing. Through the fog of tears and the lumps arising in my throat, I delivered the eulogy at Mom's funeral. I had a need to let others know who she was and that she had the assurance that she would dwell with God in eternity. I am blessed to have been her daughter and to have been given special time to get to know her before she died. For that I am grateful.

My dad had been the caregiver for Mom and when she died he was lost without her. Shortly after her death, Dad moved back to Saskatchewan. "You can take the boy away from the prairie but you can't take the prairie out of the boy." Grandpa used to say. Both my parents were born and raised in Saskatchewan. They raised all twelve of us there and retired not twenty miles from where they were born. My brother Victor took over the family farm as Mom and Dad moved into Perdue. It might have been a sense of duty or perhaps the love of driving but I spent many hours on the highway between Red Deer and Perdue. Sometimes I would drive out for coffee and return home the same day. I'm aware that this weekend is no different. At the end of this service I will get in my car and drive that too familiar road as I return to Red Deer and then to Edmonton to work in the morning. It will be a short night.

More than thirty years ago, Dad rolled the truck after a night in the pub. It was nothing short of miraculous that both he and Mom escaped without serious injury. That night he knew he needed help and promptly joined Alcoholics Anonymous. The AA program is operated as a sponsorship program and my Dad sponsored numerous people in the program over the years. Often times my visits to my parents home would be interrupted as Dad would be called out to help someone he was sponsoring avoid the pitfalls of falling off the wagon. There were times when I resented the relationship Dad developed with those he sponsored. They became his family and seemed to take what was rightfully our place. As a child, I had not had the privilege of a sober sponsor. It was a strange paradox. I was proud of my dad in his sobriety and yet I still didn't particularly like him as a person. I attended an AA birthday celebration as his guest and noted that he really didn't take ownership of being an alcoholic. Everyone else was to blame for his problems. Dad was what is sometimes referred to as a dry alcoholic. He stopped drinking but nothing much changed. He was still angry, still sarcastic and still bitter.

My dad loved to walk and in his retirement would walk twelve miles a day. He would often ask me to join him in his walks and since both of us were high energy, morning people, we enjoyed those early morning rendezvous.

I knew Dad was deeply troubled. He was not a happy man. Yet, he seemed to enjoy our conversations and often steered the conversation to God, especially after I entered the ministry. Over and over again he would ask, "Can your God really forgive me for all the horrible things I have done in my life?" I assured him that the God that I knew was a loving God, with grace to forgive all of us. "But Dad, can you forgive yourself?" I asked in return. But the question burning inside of me was, "Could I forgive him?" And what did I need to forgive him for?

On one of our walks Dad expressed his anger at me for having left the United Church to become part of the Evangelical community. "We brought you up in the United Church. Was that not good enough for you?" He inquired.

"Dad, you didn't bring me up in any church. The only time we went to church was Easter or Christmas and even that was sporadic. Then as I got a bit older I'd bum a ride with the Mainlands or the Pauls to go to service and CGIT (Christian Girls in Training). And, remember Dad, both you and Mom chose to leave the church of your parents'. Was that really any different?" I responded.

"Yes, that was different. They wouldn't allow us to get married and so we had no choice."

"Sure you had a choice and you both left. I also had a choice and felt I made the right choice for me."

"Dad, tell me what it was like for Mom to leave a religious life, to leave her church to get married and then have twelve kids?"

"I don't know. We never talked about it."

"But how could you not?" I queried. "After all, what you believe is a huge part of who you are."

"Well no, the day your mom and I got married we promised each other we would never discuss religion. And, we never did."

I knew Mom had grown up Roman Catholic. My grandmother was a devout Catholic who attended church daily whenever she could. I didn't get a sense of my Dad's parents being so connected although they were affiliated with the Church of England. It's hard for me to fathom anyone not talking about his or her faith but I guess times change. I heard some of the horror stories that accompanied my mom's exodus from the Catholic Church although I don't remember who told them. When the kids came along the local priest informed Mom that we were bastards, since the Roman Catholic Church did not recognize her marriage. She was excommunicated, informed that she was not welcome inside the Catholic Church under any circumstances, and told she would most certainly go to Hell. These had to be difficult words to hear for a young woman who, earlier in life, had considered taking vows and becoming a nun.

But times do change and ultimately my eldest sister married in the Catholic Church and both my parents and some of us "bastard" children were in attendance.

I enjoyed the walks Dad and I shared and the conversations we had. They are treasured moments. Then there are the other times.

Mom and Dad fought a lot. Late into the night we kids could hear the yelling and I remember covering my ears with a pillow to block out the sounds. It wasn't always at night. Booze was the catalyst that began many battles and brought out the worst of my dad's temper. Mom would get so frustrated as Dad drank away the money earmarked for food or clothing and Mom had to "make do." I wonder if Mom ever had a new outfit.

"The girls and I are leaving," yelled Mom as we stood by the front door, suitcases all packed and ready to go.

"You are not leaving this place," retorted my father.

I was about six-years-old at the time and this was one of many threats Mom made. She was always going to leave. But where would she go and how would she survive? She never did leave and I wonder if that was because there were so many of us. I remember only Grace and I standing at the door that night with Mom. Where were the boys? Were they going to stay with Dad? There was that rule in our house that said, "Dad was responsible for raising the boys and Mom was responsible for raising the girls." I never understood that rule. Did it apply if they split? Were we just possessions that would be apportioned and split between the two of them? Would the baby really stay with Dad? What a scary thought. Perhaps it was scary for Mom too and maybe that's why we never left. Mom often said, "I stayed for the children."

"Well don't do us any favors, thank you very much!"

I suppose Mom did raise the girls, but I think she also raised the boys, and yet I never felt close to her. With so many kids to mind there was no individual time and in particular, I felt there was never time for me. Mom was always busy being pregnant, tending to babies or being sick. She was always too busy with other things or other people.

My dad, on the other hand was mostly an embarrassment to me. I hated his drinking and swearing. I was afraid of him when he drank. He never hit me. I was one of the lucky ones and I suppose I should thank my lucky stars for that. I tried, as much as possible, to avoid Dad, especially if he'd been to town. That always meant he'd been drinking and the inevitable fighting would follow. I'd watch things from a distance and listen as the yelling got louder and louder as he and Mom fought. Sometimes I wished I could disappear. Other times I felt invisible.

If the walls of that old house could talk they would have much to say. That tattered, run down, old house couldn't even keep out the cold, but it could put on a good face and hide secrets from the outside world. Wasn't a dad someone who looked after his family? Shouldn't he know what went on within his household and wasn't he supposed to protect us from all harm? Dad had some dirty old men friends and I would retreat to my room and stay there as long as possible when they came to visit. One fellow always wanted us girls to sit on his knee and Dad couldn't see why I hated that fellow. He was a touchy, feely fellow and my skin crawled in his presence. I was filled with shame that I didn't understand. I was ashamed of being poor and simply of being a Whitfield, of being me.

But, eventually I grew up. I escaped that place that I hated so much. I graduated from high school, went to work, and then got married and moved far away. I was gone a year and a half before I went back to the farm. Relations with my parents were good over the next few years. We simply ignored past hurts and didn't talk about them. I had learned that lesson well. But, I was happily married and within four years we had two beautiful children. Life was good.

After the death of my first husband I met a wonderful man who cared for not only me, but also my children. We married in The Pas, Manitoba and my parents didn't even attend our wedding. Quite a statement, eh? I received a check in the mail as a wedding present. The check bounced. Everything old is new again.

As a child I tried hard to be the good girl. Sometimes I was more successful than others. Mostly, I tried hard to please my folks; in fact I was a pleaser and tried hard to please everyone. I did not like confrontation and there was more than enough of that to go around in our household. Although I was always told I inherited my looks from my father's family, this particular trait I inherited from my mother. For the most part, Mom was a quiet person, somewhat reserved. She would stay in the background and Dad would be the center of attention whenever we had company.

Mom was sickly much of her life. She had numerous back surgeries and between surgeries recuperated by staying in bed. Perhaps this was her way of avoiding the struggles of life. We used to joke about Mom wearing blinders. She didn't see what she didn't want to see and would never believe anything bad about her children or Dad, for that matter. Mom covered up for Dad by saying he was sick when he'd really been on a binge. My mom was an enabler. She always made excuses and covered up for Dad. I know she was afraid of his temper when he was drinking. Life certainly wasn't easy for Mom.

I feel a bit guilty as I sit at my mom's bedside, knowing that she is dying. She had been so sick for much of her life and as a teenager I believed her to be a hypochondriac. Whether there was any truth to that or not, the truth was she had certainly suffered these last seven years or so. My siblings and I planed three years in advance for our parents' fiftieth wedding anniversary. It was to be a grand event. They would renew their vows in the same church in which they were married, at St. Thomas Wesley United Church in Saskatoon. Mom doesn't remember much of that celebration. We knew something was wrong but the doctors could not seem to diagnose it correctly. Mom and Dad spent New Year's with us that year in Red Deer and Mom had a spell. She was taken to the hospital, treated with medication and released with instructions to see her family doctor as soon as they returned home. One week later Mom was diagnosed with a grapefruit sized brain tumor. She recovered from that surgery only to be diagnosed with inoperable cancer seven years later. She died in 1995 at the age of seventy-seven.

Dad died seven years later of a broken heart and loneliness (My diagnosis). In retirement he had discovered new purpose in life as the primary caregiver for Mom. He would often say, "Mom needs me and I look after her." He not only looked after her, he became adept at cooking and housecleaning and took great pride in the cleanliness of their home. He was a better housekeeper than Mom had ever been. Now, he was no longer needed and was completely lost. Life had no purpose for him and he gave up. Seven years after Mom died, Dad simply went to sleep one night and didn't wake up. My relationship with my dad was a rocky one. It was not built on solid ground. There were times when I didn't like him much and then there were other times when our relationship seemed to be good; times when he noticed me. He would display his pride in my accomplishments and I craved that recognition. It told me I was somebody.

Dad had been relatively healthy throughout his life. He had developed type-two diabetes, controlled with diet, and a few aches and pains but generally was quite medically and physically fit. He still took long daily walks. Dad never wanted to live in a nursing home and yet at age eighty-four made the decision to move into a lodge. He didn't want any of his family to have to look after him.

June 8[th,] 2002, an early morning call from my brother delivered the unexpected news that Dad had died. He had been in the Lodge less than two days. I never had the opportunity to say goodbye. Dad's remains were cremated before I completed the five-hour drive to Saskatchewan. I never understood the urgency of the immediate cremation and my need to see him in death could not be fulfilled. As a chaplain, I accompany others in this final ritual almost daily and yet could not fulfill that need with my own father. This regret weighed heavy on my heart. This pilgrimage was part of letting go of that unfulfilled need. I would say goodbye again knowing that I was someone that night at Leney Cemetery. I was one of many people gathered to pay their respects to family members who have died. I was there to take one step closer to letting go of the past and honoring my father and my mother.

The memories were strong that night. They were a mixture of the good and the bad. They were the realities of my life. The benediction was sung and the service ended.

> "Go now in peace, go now in peace.
> May the love of God surround you.
> Everywhere, everywhere, you may go."

As I left that cemetery and headed for home, I was at peace.

Summary

It was difficult to write these stories and yet there was a sense of freedom as I wrote. Perhaps these stories have spoken to you. It is my hope that my stories will convey the message, to all who read them, that their stories are important, too, and need to be told. The following chapter is my reflection on my heuristic self-search inquiry of researching and exploring my healing journey through story.

CHAPTER FIVE

HEURISTIC REFLECTION

The heuristic process is a way of being informed, a way of knowing. Whatever presents itself in the consciousness of the investigator as perception, sense, intuition, or knowledge represents an invitation for further elucidation (Moustakas 10).

Introduction

In this chapter I will share my reflections on the six phases of heuristic self-search inquiry in response to my question, "What is the experience of healing as revealed through story?" I look at two metaphors that speak to my experience and reflect on the themes that are prominent throughout the process. I reflect on the connections between healing and story throughout my self-search inquiry as I seek to highlight those insights I have gleaned.

Story is not only who I am, it is what I do. As a chaplain in a hospital I bring an aspect of holistic healing to a multi-disciplinary setting and so my passionate interest in the connection between story and healing comes naturally. What didn't come naturally was a burning passion to discover how those elements combined in *my own* journey. The interest was always present. The shift to self-search inquiry was divine intervention. The initial engagement was that process of putting the question into proper perspective to allow me to "encounter myself in a way that is autobiographical and touches significant relationships within my social context" (Sela-Smith 64).

Reflection on the immersion phase, in which I became one with my question, will give the reader insight into what it was like for me to go back in time and revisit memories from the past. Incubation allowed those experiences to germinate, to foster new growth within my spirit and to illuminate my vision as transformation and new understanding took place. Through explication I entered into a process of seeking greater understanding and awareness. The research culminated in a creative synthesis that rounded out the dissertation and the remaining chapters. The phases were not mutually exclusive, but rather merged together in a natural flow as I revisited, reflected, wrote, reflected and wrote again as demonstrated by my diagram, *Data Gathering & Reflection Process* (32). Each phase invited interaction and further reflection either culminating in healing and transformation or opening the doors for future possibility.

This heuristic self-search inquiry has very much been that process described by Moustakas and quoted at the beginning of this chapter. It is a way of being informed, a way of knowing myself by listening to the stories within and then giving voice and space for them to unfold. In challenging, confronting, doubting and then acknowledging, accepting and reframing my experiences space is created for healing and growth. All of this became data for reflection throughout the research process. When "experience, feeling and meaning joined together to form new pictures of my world and new ways to navigate that world" (Sela-Smith 69) my data spoke to my soul and became tacit knowledge in which I *knew* things differently.

Recurring themes such as resistance, defensiveness, shame and guilt, the need to prove myself, self-sabotage, self-acceptance, listening to myself, believing in myself, accepting the truth of my own story and rediscovering God were predominant throughout my life and were important aspects of my self-search inquiry as I sought to respond to my question, "What is the experience of healing as revealed through story?" Each of these themes is evident in various ways in the stories I share in chapter four and the entire research process. In the exploration of my own healing and the role of story in that healing I have connected my experience with the available literature.

Metaphorically Speaking

As I entered this reflection on healing I remembered two movies, which struck me as particularly powerful metaphors. The first was a story by Otto Klement, which became the foundation of the movie Fantastic Voyage. The voyage, not unlike my own inner healing journey, is indeed both incredible and fantastic. As I watched the movie for a second time the analogy became clearer. The actors who became miniscule and traveled inside the blood stream to the brain to do a healing work encountered resistance and many hurdles. Revisiting stages of my life in this dissertation process has brought me to places of resistance and hurdles. Like one of the doctors in the movie, I have been tempted to turn back, to sabotage the journey and give up. In the movie there were those who chose to continue on, to overcome each hurdle and reach the final destination. I choose (present tense) to reach the final destination, to finish the race set before me and in the end to be able to say as the writer of Hebrews so eloquently put it, "therefore, since we have so great a cloud of witnesses surrounding us, let us also lay aside every encumbrance, and the sin which so easily entangles us, and *let us run with endurance the race that is set before us*" (*Emphasis added* Hebrews 12:1).

The second movie is a film, Back to the Future, in which Marty Fly, played by Canadian actor Michael J. Fox, is accidentally spirited back in time by way of a time machine. He goes back in time thirty years to a time before he was born. He learns his family history by being a part of it. This dissertation journey has catapulted me back in time to relive my own history. My time machine has been my memory, my heart and my pen. Marty tries to manipulate the events in the past to cement his future, while I try to utilize my history to grow, to heal and then move forward in confidence and a sense of well-being.

The Process of Heuristic Self-Search Inquiry

The process of heuristic self-search inquiry is not linear and so it is difficult, if not impossible, to simply look at the process step-by-step. The key component of Sela-Smith's approach that grabbed my attention was "resistance" in which I as the researcher had to acknowledge "resistance to feeling in the reconnection with the *I-who-feels*" (85). The ability to move beyond resistance is essential to self-search inquiry. I discovered it was not entirely possible to stay in the feelings but rather I found myself moving in and out from the "*I-who-feels*" (57) to the *I-who-observes*. As I reflected on my own resistance I became aware that part of me did not want to revisit my pain-filled experiences. The incest and alcoholism were parts of my past that I wanted to keep hidden. The fact that I can't remember a whole lot about my brother who was the perpetrator of that incest, tells me there is still resistance to going there. Whitfield tells us "many adult children of alcoholic, troubled or dysfunctional families cannot remember up to 75% of their childhood experiences" (101). I still shudder at the memories of how dirty and unworthy I felt. I am not able to totally be the "*I-who-feels*" (Sela-Smith 57). There is a measure of healing in my ability to acknowledge and claim my own reality in the experience.

Initially I began by writing other peoples' stories. There was perhaps a safety element in attempting to tell the stories of others. I could look at the healing aspects of story from a distance. Although I was involved in these stories, it was at a different level and I wasn't exposed. There was an element of emotional investment but I was probably the opposite of what Sela-Smith would refer to as the "*I-who-feels*" (57). I was merely the *I-who-observes* as the stories touched me without risking my own transparency and vulnerability.

In retrospect, I was confronted with my own humanity and subconscious fear of the vulnerability and exposure in that inward gaze at my own stories. Herbert Anderson and Edward Foley remind me of the power of storytelling. As I read their account of the women of Rwanda and how they were healed of sleeplessness as, one-by-one, they told their stories of the carnage of civil war (*Mighty Stories, Dangerous Rituals* 3), I am taken back to the carnage at ground zero in New York City, post 9/11, where I witnessed firsthand the power of storytelling. Each survivor, each worker, had a story and a need to tell it. As a chaplain I was privileged to be the conduit to supply that listening ear. But there is a difference in listening to, or writing the stories of others and peering deep within my soul to disclose that, which has been hidden for so long. I, like those women of Rwanda, had learned the importance of keeping secrets.

My question, "what is the experience of healing as revealed through story?" first seeded itself in my heart and then germinated in my soul. My dissertation shifted from an external story to my internal story. I became immersed in a process, which was simultaneously exhilarating and scary. It was both life-giving and life-draining. The gamut of emotions was overwhelming and, like a roller-coaster ride at a country fair, I was tossed 'hither and yon.' My stomach ached and I felt nauseous knowing I could not get off the ride. The poetic words of Frederick Buechner attest to the experience of becoming one with my question:

> Loving, living and alone
> I stood as silent as a stone
> Until within the corner of my ring
> I found myself, and that was everything (*The Sacred Journey* 89).

In finding myself, and accepting who I am, there is recognition of the importance of my story and the possibility to reframe my experiences seen in light of new discoveries. Both Buechner and Paul stress the importance of recognizing that we matter. Paul then encourages us to "value your own story through writing. What you can uniquely write will benefit you and bless others, because you matter and your story matters" (16) while Buechner writes of the importance of finding oneself.

> And although I think I knew even then that finding that self and being that self and protecting and nurturing and enjoying that self was not the "everything" I called it in the poem, by and large it was everything that, to me, really mattered (91).

Heuristic self-search inquiry demands that I search for myself; that I look inward, that I re-member, and that I reflect and remain open to new insights and learning. I have spent much time in the immersion stage. It is in this stage that I literally lived the question. Sela-Smith claims,

> The researcher is able to become intimately involved in the question ... to live the question and grow in knowledge and understanding... It (the question) appears to have a power that draws the image of the question everywhere in the researcher's life experience (65).

I found, much to my surprise that everything in my daily life began to speak directly to me with pronounced significance in a manner that could not be ignored. I was immersed in the process. My question became an inseparable part of me. It was as though everything and everyone knew I was on this quest and all I had to do was tune in. The importance of story was being emphasized in every aspect of my life. At work I was asked to take the lead in our Caritas Health Group *Sacred Story Initiative,* in which we are soliciting healing stories from staff, patients, and family members for a book to be published next year. I attended a seminar on hope during which we were encouraged to write our stories with new vision. One Sunday our pastor reminded us that we are more than conquerors. We are overcomers, who are completely forgiven and are perfect in God's sight. I heard, with new insight that the renewal of our minds refers to a change in how we see ourselves. It is both knowing and believing who we are in Christ and living out of that. Colleagues, general conversations, Sunday sermons, staff meetings, and even my radio, as I traveled back and forth to work on a daily basis, spoke directly into my life and into my healing journey. I began to understand what it was to be totally in the immersion stage of my research. I heard what I needed to hear and saw God's hand in it all.

I would stay in the feelings and allow the journey to unfold as it would. And yet, that was difficult. It was difficult at times to write, to reveal my story, to go back in time and attempt to relive the experience. I experienced writer's block and resistance. There were times when I didn't want to write and times when I literally couldn't. Parts of my story confronted me and I had to force myself to stay in the moment and then go forward, resisting temptation to run. I almost wished the moral ethicist I had contracted to journey along side me would help me to discover that morally I must avoid telling certain aspects of my story. But in the long run I had to face the music and get real with myself.

I have looked deep into my soul and questioned my own motives around writing. Was I doing this strictly for a dissertation or were there deeper reasons? When I started on this "fantastic voyage" I promised myself that I would be true to the process. As I reflect back on the metaphor of the movie Fantastic Voyage, I stated that, "like one of the Doctors in the movie I have been tempted to turn back, to sabotage the journey and give up" (99). *Self-sabotage* is another of those themes that play out on the stage of my life. As I reflect I wonder if at least part of the answer to a question posed by one of my committee members as he wanted to know if there was an element of escapism for me as I respond to disasters in various parts of the world. In reflection I believe I do this not only to respond to those in need but also to escape the uncomfortable challenges in my life. As I neared the end of this dissertation I became aware that part of me did not want to finish it. I just wanted to go away and scrap it all. Resistance, avoidance and self-sabotage were all at play. I wanted to give in and give up. That surely would have sabotaged my dissertation and prevented revealing the secrets I would still rather keep hidden. It is not easy to give up the pretense of being that television situation comedy family, "The Brady Bunch" from the early seventies, and recognize the reality of the poor dysfunctional Whitfield family.

Another theme that arises throughout my life, my stories and my reflection is my *defensive attitude*. It was ingrained in me as a child and was a survival technique. Although my defense mechanisms served me well in my growing up years, I realize that it is difficult to be simultaneously vulnerable and defensive. Defensiveness helped me to put on the veil of secrecy and build a wall of protection around my feelings and emotions. Defensiveness and resistance go hand-in-hand. Part of not wanting to tell my stories, comes from wanting to protect our family name. (That is so like my father!) I don't want the reality of a dysfunctional family. I want the "white picket fence" and "they lived happily ever-after." I want my memories to be the fantasies I lived in my childhood. Oh, how I wished that were so, but it is not.

Charles Whitfield has helped me understand my need to "Protect the parents and thus block healing" (102). I recognize myself in his words as he outlines the ways we do this with the following chart reprinted from *Healing the Child Within* (102).

Answers, Approaches and Strategies Often Used
to Protect the Parents (and thus Block Healing)

Category	Frequently Heard
1) Outright denial	"My childhood was fine."
2) Appeasing: "Yes, but . . .,	"It happened but . . . they (my parents) did their best."
3) Viewing pain of the trauma as a fantasy	"It really didn't happen that way."
4) Fourth Commandment	"God will be angry at me. It just isn't right."
5) Unconscious fear of rejection	"If I express my rage, they won't love me."
6) Fear of the unknown	Something really bad will happen. I might hurt someone, or they might hurt me."
7) Accepting the Blame	"I'm the bad one."
8) Forgiving the parents	"I'll just forgive them" or "I've already forgiven them."
9) Attacking the person who suggests doing recovery work	"You're bad for suggesting that I express my hurt and rage or that my parents could have been bad."

Most of the strategies were part of my repertoire of coping mechanisms. I can distinctly hear my voice, in my memory, declaring, "my childhood was fine, "it really didn't happen," and "it happened, but they (my parents) did their best." These "knee jerk reactions were how I survived. They were my defenses.

Whitfield explores the meaning of the commandment "to honor thy father and thy mother" (Exodus 20:12 AV). He says,

> It is difficult to decipher or interpret exactly what the word "honor" means…
> Over the centuries, it has been interpreted by most *parents* to mean "no back
> talk" and other such stifling messages to the child" (103).

In reflection I realize this was exactly what it meant to honour my parents. It also meant to "do as I say, not as I do" and to obey without question. As children we were to be "seen and not heard." For me I preferred to be neither seen nor heard. I believe it was providential that I named the segment of my journey involving my parents, "Honor thy Father and thy Mother." Through both writing and reflecting on those experiences I have been able to reframe not only the experiences themselves but also the meaning of honor. In accepting and understanding myself more fully I am able to view my parents through a different lens, come to a greater understanding of them as persons and realize that life was not easy for them. We learn our coping skills from observation of our parents and unless we are fortunate enough to recognize our own woundedness and take steps to change our attitudes and behaviours, we continue the cycle. My parents had their own coping skills and without malice or denial I can say I truly believe they tried their best to cope with raising twelve children within very limited means. I do not make this statement out of "cheap forgiveness," nor from the defensive stance reflected in Whitfield's chart. After deep soul-searching and immersion in the process of this research I removed many roadblocks and came to the path of healing. As I journey on this path I reflect further on those coping mechanisms that played such an important role in my life.

> Survivors are by necessity co-dependents. We use many coping skills and ego
> defenses to do this… while these defenses are functional in our dysfunctional
> family, they tend to work poorly for us as adults (60).

These roadblocks are now invitations to healing and growth. Resistance lingers still and I found myself asking who might read my stories and would my truth bring harm or hurt to anyone else? After all, my stories are not mine alone. I wondered aloud,

> *Realistically, who would read my dissertation? Part of me hoped that it would be limited to my committee, an external reader and perhaps the head of the doctor of ministry program. I am faced with the horrible truth that part of me did not wish to see this dissertation to fruition. If I never completed it then I wouldn't have to wonder who might read it. There would be no possible fallout or damage that could be inflicted on others. Mostly, I would not have to reveal all my hidden memories. I wished I had a pleasant story to write. But, life is what it is and so this is my story and it does need to be told* (Personal journal notes).

To reflect on the experience of healing as revealed through my story it was necessary for me to not only write my stories, but it was essential that I listen to what they say to me as I read them to myself. Eugene Kennedy said,

> Pause to listen and what would we hear? We would hear the messages of our feelings, the very messages we so often ignore or to which we pay little attention. There is so much noise in life that they are sometimes drowned out. And we are often in such a hurry to do this or that that we do not listen at all. These messages are always there, however, and all we need is some time and a quiet place in which to listen to them (*If You Really Knew Me Would You Still Like Me?* (80-81).

I hear the messages of my feelings. I hear the denial of abuse. I *hear* the resistance I feel at the thoughts of exposing my family secrets. I wonder if is it possible that while there may be truth in Kennedy's words, there is also some truth that the same "noise" affects all living beings and that at times we use it to avoid facing our own truth? Do I hurry to avoid the vulnerability of hearing myself? I fill everyday with too many commitments, too many meetings that often leave no time to sit and reflect. I fear the pain of the stories that can heal and so I avoid them. In *resistance* I move with the noise and even though I know I need time and a quiet place in which to listen, the truth is, I don't want to listen. The words, "Be still

and know ... (Psalm 46:10), echo in my ears but it is hard for me to be still and listen.

I have lived my life in a whirlwind of activity, perhaps hoping to ignore those

messages of my feelings. The theme that fits well here is that of *avoidance*. In my

whirlwind of activity I keep myself so busy that I don't have time to be still and listen. "Oh,

I'm a little hyper," I would declare, never wanting to take time to listen to that still, small

voice within. I was afraid of what it would say, and I knew with certainty that if ever you

really knew me, you wouldn't like me. Behind the veil that hid my face were all my secret

fears and insecurities. I could create my own image and be brave in the face of adversity. As

a child I spent much time reading and fantasizing on the life I *should* have had. This, too,

was my way of avoiding the reality of my everyday life. Like Orual in, *Till We Have Faces,*

I found strength in my veil. It was my defense against the world. Orual says, 'the best story

was that I had no face at all; if you stripped off my veil you'd find emptiness" (C. S. Lewis

228). There's a hollow feeling that echoes inside me as those words penetrate my soul.

They read me well. Today I can remove my veil and move beyond that emptiness and so I

write my stories and in reflection allow them to change me and reveal my face.

Contrary to my belief that if you really knew me you wouldn't like me, author Susan

Paul quite boldly declares that "You matter and your story matters" (22). She then asks and

answers the question,

> Why write? Because God writes. All life is founded by God and his
> marvelous creativity... *God writes his story*. There is vast evidence in the
> Bible that God wants the story of his interaction with people to be written
> down. The prophets were told to write down what they experienced and their
> messages from God because it mattered to God that his word and his story be
> preserved for future generations (*Your Story Matters* 22).

If my story matters then I must tell it. I owe it to my family, to God, to the greater

community and to myself. I was a daydreamer and I imagined my story to be much different

than it actually was. But my story is important and all the experiences within that story

combine to make me who I am.

> Made in God's image ("a little higher that the angels" the Bible says) *you* are
> unique. No one else has your fingerprints or DNA code, and *no one else has*
> *your story* (Paul 11).

These words reinforce the need to tell my story. Although my story is

uniquely mine, it is not mine alone and so I tell it not only for my own healing but, for the

benefit of others as I heed the advice of Paul.

> Writing down who we are-where we come from, what our life has been like
> and what it is right now-is valuable in creating new dialogues among families,
> friends and future generations (109).

These words echo my experience. As I wrote, my sisters often became the ears to

hear and as we talked, we reminisced and shared our common stories. We cried together and

laughed together and the possibility for the healing journey to expand to other family

members opened up. As I wrote, it was my intention to create new dialogue, first of all

within myself as I reframed the experiences in ways that allowed me to remove myself from

being responsible for my own abuse. There is both power and healing in claiming this

freedom. This power allows me to create new dialogue in my personal life with family,

friends and future generations and then in the context of my ministry. Although Egnew's

article was written in relation to the medical community it sites wisdom that transcends

disciplinary boundaries and can readily be connected to the community at large. He quotes

Imui as describing healing as occurring in contexts of "real persons in connection with other

real persons" (4) and claims, "Life narratives are social constructions, stories fashioned in connection with others" (4). As I reinterpret my life through my stories there is healing and I am drawn anew into community with others.

I resonate with the words of Julie Nelson Lahmeyer, nurse and pastor's wife, from Auburn Washington, who endorses *Your Story Matters,* with the following words "It is healing for me to think about how my story matters and it has given me new energy for ministry and relationships" (2). Not only is there healing in the dawning realization that my stories matter but further, as I am able to give voice to my stories and lay them out, to expose them for what they are, they lose their power over me. The balance of power shifts and I am no longer caught in the secrecy. I am free to take control of elements of healing in my own life.

Some of my stories were quite "safe" and were simply part of my own healing experience. Others took me to places I would rather not have gone. Going back in time to the death of my first husband made me look again at my own grief and loss. I am good at teaching about grief and loss and I can 'talk a good talk' as I minister to those going through the experience. I believe God works through my experience and I can relate to others who are suffering loss partly because I've been there. I am more compassionate and understanding. I have more patience and while some of that may be attributed to maturity, there is also the knowledge that I am good at what I do because of a combination of God's grace and life's experience.

One of the most important lessons of chaplaincy is the need to deal with one's own *stuff.* If we are stuck in our own grief or pain, we cannot help others. I know, on a personal level, I have dealt with grief in healthy ways, through groups, through counseling, and through surrounding myself with those to whom I hold myself accountable. This self-search inquiry process has confirmed for me that grief is not a one time, *get over it*, thing. It is a life-long process and those intense moments of grief can return without warning. Yesterday returns with a vengeance to say, "I'm still a part of you, deal with me." Healing demands a great deal from us. It ultimately calls forth a letting go and then given space, time and opportunity, healing happens.

Writing the Healing Journey

I chose several segments of my life that represented the potential for healing. In the initial engagement phase, as I contemplated embarking on this journey, I reflected on those things that I am passionate about. I am intensely interested in issues around death, dying and grief. I am passionate in my concern and care for the marginalized and disadvantaged in our society. This has led me into the ministry of chaplaincy in which I journey with and support others in the difficult times in their lives. In self-dialogue and inner search I encountered myself, and my autobiography within this context. As my question formed and lingered within me it revealed that I had unresolved issues around death, dying and grief. I was the marginalized and the disadvantaged and needed to explore those aspects of my life that created those realities. "Telling our story is a powerful act in discovering and healing our child within" (Whitfield 96). I am getting to know myself more deeply in writing, telling, listening and reflecting on my stories.

A visit to our old family farm with my grandson and then later by myself afforded me the opportunity to put my memories in perspective and recognize the aspects of my childhood that were joyous along with the painful memories. Along with that change in perception came a healing of memories. I no longer cringe when I think of the farm.

As I began to put pen to paper I discovered that it was a difficult challenge. I could speak to trusted friends or colleagues within a margin of safety and yet discovered that at times it was nearly impossible to write. *Writing as a Way of Healing* has served as a great encouragement and guide in my process. DeSalvo says, "The act of writing about something painful can help right a wrong that has been done to you" (10). Writing has been, for me, a way of releasing pent up emotions and a way of letting go of the past. As I reach inside, grab hold of the pain and place it on the paper, there is a sense of healing. That sense of healing is difficult to describe. It is like having an infection and having it lanced. The pressure is released and as the infection oozes out and the pain is relieved. Writing is an aid to healing. It is not a miraculous instantaneous cure all.

DeSalvo stresses the importance of "learning how to care for ourselves as we embark upon complex but significant writing so that we can benefit from the healing potential of telling our stories" (94).

As I wrote my stories and entered into dialogue with them, part of my self-care was to physically drive back to the location of the experience. I love to drive and time in my car is therapeutic for me. When I am in my car it is impossible for me to busy myself with other activities and I enter into a sanctuary where I listen and reflect. I drove to Saskatchewan a number of times as I wrote "Through the Eyes of a Child," "The Teenage Years," and "Honor thy Father and thy Mother." I drove to Thompson, Manitoba as I wrote Memories. Other things I did to care for myself included going to a retreat center for one month so that I could concentrate on writing, reflecting and being in the presence of God. It was wintertime and I walked on the frozen lake for hours seeking discernment and wisdom.

As I began to write I chose the path of least resistance. Perhaps it was divine intervention but the first story I wrote, although it represented a specific, significant healing, was lighter and not as heart wrenching in the writing. I didn't feel as exposed as I imagined I would with some of the other stories. But in being true to the process I was determined to do what needed to be done.

I reflected on the tremendous courage of writers like Dave Pelzer, who shared the horrendous experience of his childhood in *A Child Called It.* The healing in his life is evident as the reader follows his life journey through to *The Lost Boy,* and *A Man Called Dave,* when after extreme abuse, at the hands of his mother, he claims his own identity as a man. He survived abuses almost beyond comprehension. I wept as I read his story and almost felt ashamed of even expressing a desire to use the term abuse in my own experience. I found myself devaluing and denigrating my own experience. But the reality was that my childhood was dysfunctional. It was my experience and was extremely personal to me. In reflection I can admit and accept that reality and know that it was wrong. The healing aspect of revisiting, writing and reflecting comes from admitting and accepting that reality along with the pain and knowledge of how very wrong it was and that it was not my fault. In retrospect I also see that life was not all bad and that all of my experiences are part and parcel of the strength, courage, and character of who I am. I made decisions in my life based on those experiences.

In reflection, I realize that the stories for my healing journey, as I first anticipated writing them, did not happen. I had neatly mapped out the order but with the passage of time, immersion and the entire heuristic research methodology and self-search inquiry, the process itself claimed space and took an unexpected turn.

My recorded journey claimed its own order, not predetermined by my rational thought process but rather by what I believe to be a combination of prayerful discernment and divine intervention. In the final analysis, I believe God has directed my path and I revealed what I needed to share.

"Be still and know that I am God" (Psalm 46:10) is a scripture passage that keeps speaking into my life. Being still is not easy for me and demands obedience to a call to allow space for God and to provide a listening ear to hear. "He, who has ears to hear, let him hear" (Mark 4:9). To hear, to really hear, not only with my ears, but also with my heart it is sometimes necessary to be still to hear and understand what is being said. As I read "Honor thy Father and Thy Mother" to my younger sister I listened to the story and was able to pause and reflect on our parents' lives. What experiences did they have as children? Were their families dysfunctional? In knowing some of their stories, I imagined the difficulties they encountered and I listened with new insight to my story.

I have appreciated the wisdom expressed in *Healing the Child Within*, which has helped me to go to greater depths of understanding. Whitfield, along with others, has been a tremendous resource as I have struggled to make sense of my own experience, not in comparison to the experiences of others, but rather seeking perspective on where they fit in the totality of my life. Experiences that I have previously chosen not to look at, not to recognize as part of the fabric of my life have taken on new significance. Feelings of guilt and shame have claimed space in my life and have inhibited my healing process. Guilt is feeling wrongness of action, while shame is feeling wrongness of being. I made a mistake versus I am a mistake. This is a powerful distinction. "I am a mistake" was often how I felt as a child. This was compounded by the feelings that there was no room for me and I really wasn't wanted and didn't belong. The slap my mother administered when I accusingly asked whether she had ever heard of birth control suggests that she may never have "wanted" or planned to have all twelve of us. This reinforced the negative messages, such as "I wish you'd never been born" "stupid" "never good enough." Add to those the "poor Whitfield brats" felt by the actions of well-meaning neighbors as they dropped off their old hand-me-downs and seemed to look down their noses at us. Whitfield suggested that "Our shame seems to come from what we do with the negative messages, negative affirmations, beliefs and rules that we hear as we grow up" (46). What I did was to reinforce the negative messages and added a few more as I repeated them over and over again to myself. The rules in our household were simple; just do as I say, not as I do, respect your elders, obey your parents and do not air our dirty laundry in public. There was no rationale for the messages or the rules and they contributed to the dysfunction in our household. In reading and reflection I know these old tapes do not identify me. Deepak Chopra says, "The tormentor today is myself left over from yesterday" (*Healing from the Heart* 133). I do not want to be left-over, that is too much like hand-me-down. And so I replace the old tapes by moving forward and changing the tune to create a new song for myself.

Maddix and Soles share the story of a nursing home resident who, after a pilgrimage to Lourdes in southwest France, when asked by a student if she had been cured at Lourdes responded, "No, but I have come to a new meaning in my life and I am prepared to go on with the next stage"(22). This was reflective of my healing journey throughout this dissertation process.

The Continuing Journey

This dissertation has been part of my healing journey as throughout the process there have been many frustrations, feelings of betrayal, anger, and despair. Ultimately there has been healing and growth and the learning process has been rich and rewarding.

I have learned to hold material things more lightly as a result of having spent three and one half months in Africa, training chaplains and then more recently, three weeks assisting Hurricane Katrina victims in Mississippi in the midst of my studies. In reflection I noted that on my return from these mission trips I dealt with my perceived materialism by giving away possessions. But *letting go* is bigger than that; it is much more than letting go of materialism. It is recognizing that I am not perfect, I am not superwoman and I am not in control of all things in my life. It is releasing preconceived ideas, reliving my story and allowing it to unfold anew.

Dr. Richard LaPlante's death had a tremendous impact on my life and my program. LaPlante, former head of the Doctor of Ministry program, had been my encouragement as I entered St. Stephen's college and struggled with differing theologies. At one point, early in the process, I was feeling discouraged and overwhelmed. As I met with LaPlante I shared my frustrations and expressed my desire to withdraw from the program. LaPlante encouraged me to continue on and shared with me that as he, a Roman Catholic came to St. Stephen's, his strength and groundedness in his own faith deepened. His words of wisdom to me were: "It would be my hope that St. Stephen's would make you a better Pentecostal, not that they would make you a liberal theologian." I left his office that day with new resolve to complete the journey unfolding before me. So, in retrospect, am I a better Pentecostal and what does that look like? I do know that I am more firmly grounded in my faith and thus can minister ecumenically in my role as hospital chaplain.

This dissertation has changed considerably from the original plan drafted back in the year 2000. Not only has the plan changed, my entire doctoral committee has changed. Not one member of the committee, who are alongside me today as I enter the final phases towards completion, was originally on my committee. While I am grateful for everyone who has been part of the process, that reality has been frustrating.

Two years ago, as I prepared to go to Africa at the invitation of both the Ministry of Health and the Baptist Conference, as a visiting professor to train chaplains within the Health care System, I was euphoric. I had completed my dissertation draft and it was in the hands of my committee. I was assured that it would go to an external reader early in the New Year. Something changed. By mid February I e-mailed the person acting as liaison on my committee asking if my dissertation had been forwarded to the external reader. In place of a reply from my liaison, I got an e-mail from the new Head of the Doctor of Ministry program telling me that my dissertation would not be forwarded to the external reader and that my committee would meet with me on my return. No one was prepared to talk to me until then. My plans for convocation in 2003 were dashed. I was devastated. This information came totally out of left field. I felt betrayed. I was thousands of miles away from home and all my support systems. I had no one to talk to. I didn't understand how this could be happening. I felt as though I was drowning. I did not know what to do with this new information. I tried to put it out of my mind but that did not prove to be very successful. My time in Cameroon was only half over. I still had much work to do and was in the process of writing a manual for chaplaincy training in Africa. I was to present it before returning to Canada. I buried myself in my work determined not to let the devastating news regarding my dissertation destroy me or derail my work in Cameroon. It was around this time that I got very sick and subsequently came to realize that I had to focus on my mission there and let go of the horrible feeling of failure.

This was the beginning of a huge learning curve and a lesson in letting go and allowing the process to happen. I found strength as the solitude of illness pulled me into intense prayer and reliance on God as my strength and my comfort. I remember, amidst hallucinations in my delirium, feeling as though I were being attacked by strange beings and calling out to God. Although I was under a doctor's care, I was living by myself and spent two fitful nights, afraid to go to sleep, drifting in and out of consciousness and feeling as though I was losing my mind. I have never felt so vulnerable or so alone. I did not want to die in Africa. I just kept calling on the name of Jesus to help me. This experience brought me to a place, during my recovery, of deep reflection on what is truly important to me in life. I thought of family and knew the love and relationships of those I hold dear were the most important things in my life. My faith had sustained me. God brought me through this difficult time and I knew beyond a shadow of a doubt that with God's help I could face whatever the future held.

Shortly after arriving back in Canada my dissertation committee, with the exception of one member, disbanded. I felt as though I had taken five steps forward, the number of chapters in my dissertation, and then six steps back. Six steps back took me to beginning again with a new design.

Initially I was completing my doctorate in the art modality and writing stories of people with whom I had journeyed. The art modality, itself, seemed to present a problem. I understand that the introduction of the art modality had been LaPlante's initiative and now with him gone, there was a lack of clarity on what the expectations were from the college point of view.

There was another possibility I had to face. Perhaps the work I had done up to now, really was not at a doctoral level. Writing a doctoral dissertation is tough work. A doctorate differs from a Master's program in that it combines the academic and the experiential in an integrative learning style. My committee had undergone several changes. That should have been a clue to me. Were my previous committee members trying to direct me and was I so focused on my own agenda that I was blind to their direction? Was that why my committee had changed numerous times? Did they find it impossible to work with me and even more impossible to communicate that reality to me? Was that why the newly appointed head of the Doctoral Studies had the responsibility of informing me of decisions of the committee? Although I felt abandoned and betrayed, my own stubbornness and inability to hear were stumbling blocks that I didn't want to recognize.

Now, I was faced with a monumental decision. I was tempted to withdraw from the process and knew I would have been in good company. Ric had given us statistics at one point that showed that less than forty percent of those beginning a doctorate ever complete it. I had spent three years of my life becoming absorbed in this process. I found myself questioning why I was doing this at this stage of my life. What difference would having a doctorate really mean to me? Was I willing to do whatever was needed to achieve this goal? The truth was there was not a simple answer. My husband calls me a perennial student. I have studied most of my life and the reality is that in many ways, I love the challenge and I love to learn. The other reality is that while there is a drivenness about me that demands much of myself, sometimes that drivenness can be unrealistic.

A new committee was struck and they were all in agreement. They were in this for the long haul and willing to go the distance. But they were demanding and the results were that my entire focus changed. It is not easy to embark on a self-search inquiry in which it feels as though I have exposed my life to strangers for them to examine it and put a stamp of approval, or disapproval, on it. I recognize that committee approval is not on my life itself but rather on the skill of writing in such a manner that readers will recognize their lives in my stories. But it is difficult to separate the writing from the experience and that too is part of the learning.

Once the decision to continue had been made, there was no turning back and the process has been a tremendous eye opener for me. I can put things in perspective and know that my own healing journey will continue long after this dissertation is completed, unless I should die in the meanwhile, although even then maybe the healing continues as "death is swallowed up in victory" (1 Corinthians15:54).

The Challenges

Throughout this dissertation process I was challenged to look closely at who I am and why I do what I do. In refection it seems important to give space to that part of the journey as it led to revelation and insight into self-understanding.

I was asked, at one particularly difficult time, if perhaps everything that was transpiring throughout the process "was part of the healing journey." I'm a bit ashamed as I reflect on my reaction at the time. I was taken aback by the question and quite indignant in my response. The rejection of my doctoral work was too close. My head knew it was not rejection of my person, but my heart did not. I was not at a place wherein I was able to separate my work from my person. If what I was doing was rejected, it seemed to reflect on me as a person and mean that I was not acceptable. I felt like a failure. In reflection I realized that this was one of those old tapes, of "not being good enough" being played over again. In prayerful discernment I have been able to look to the bigger picture and listen to advice and then determine for myself what direction I need to go. I believe God's hand has been directing the process and the direction of my dissertation as it eventually unfolded into being my own healing journey through story, not only for my benefit but for the benefit of others needing encouragement. There was rich insight and revelation as I came to a deeper understanding of myself and allow that to absorb in my heart and in my soul.

I was challenged to look at "Why do you do what you do? Why do you feel called to respond to invitations to serve in Africa, Mississippi, New York, and other places?"

My response was, "I do this because it is my way of giving back, of helping the hurting people in the world. I have a sense of call in responding to needs, either through the Red Cross or through mission work through my church or other organizations. I have a need to reach out and help others and be part of a more global community."

"Yes, but is there something more? Is there a part in which this becomes an escape for you?"

I pondered his question and I believe, in reflection, there is probably at least an element of truth in the desire to escape. I know that I have a heart for missions. I love to travel and I love to be in the midst of people from other areas of the world. I do not have a need to travel first class, nor to stay in fancy hotels. I can live and work amidst disaster and poverty wherever I am called to go. I believe my growing up was preparation for my functioning abilities in less prosperous areas of the world, and maybe was instrumental in developing within me a heart for the underprivileged. In reflection I also recognize my desire to escape the reality of facing again the painful times in my life and exposing those realities for others to see. I have run before. I make snap decisions and act on those in the immediacy of the moment. Partly that is who I am, but there is more to it than that. I recall, very soon after my husband died, I made the decision to move to another town and go back to school. Less than two months after he died, my two children and I had relocated and I was back in school full time. Was an irrational part of me trying to establish some normalcy by changing our lives completely? Was this part of my denial? Was it an escape? Perhaps! As this dissertation drew to a close I knew that a part of me did not want to finish it. I did not want my stories printed. I wanted to escape and run away. Noewen says, "The answer to your question is hidden in your heart" (35). So, the answer to the question, "Why do I do what I do?" is two-fold. I do what I do both to escape and to respond to a sense of call to reach out and help those in need.

As I wrote my research notes and submitted them I was challenged to reflect on why I wrote in the passive tense. Again there are a couple of reasons for this. The first one is probably more surface and I would say that part of the reason I wrote in the passive tense was that it is a habit that I practice daily. As I chart, I am expected to record in the passive tense. In written notes we do not use our names or the names of patient's. The deeper reason is that hesitancy around claiming my stories knowing they are being put out there for others to read. I feel a little bit like I imagine my patient's must feel as they speak of loosing all sense of privacy on entering hospital. I have been exposed as surely as if I were wearing one of those awful hospital gowns that hide nothing.

These challenges have encouraged me to reflect on who I am. Reflecting on the questions may not, in and of itself, change things but I know that I will continue the quest to understand myself more completely. Each opportunity for self-search and reflection opens the doors for greater awareness, understanding and transformation. As I trust the process and allow it to unfold I am enriched.

Summary

In summary of heuristic research I have looked at key concepts in the literature along with insights I have gained in conducting the research and those insights which have been reinforced for me in the process.

The following key concepts in the literature support my research findings:

- Sela-Smith includes resistance as one of the key components of her self-search inquiry. She says we need to stay in our feelings to move beyond resistance (85)

- Paul tells us our stories matter and we have both a need and a responsibility to tell our stories (22)

- Buechner stresses the importance of "finding oneself" (91)

- Anderson & Foley attest to the healing power of story (3)

- Whitfield outlines how, in dysfunctional families, children protect themselves by "Protecting the parents and blocking healing" (102)

- Kennedy calls us to listen to ourselves and the messages of our feelings (80-81)

- Whitfield states that telling our story is a powerful act in discovering and healing our child within (96)

- DeSalvo stresses the importance of self-care in order to benefit from the healing potential of telling our stories (94)

- Scripture tells us to "Be still and know… (Psalm 46:10).

I have gained some new insights which I see as gifts, while other insights are not new to me but have been reinterpreted, enriched and reinforced by my research process.

Gifts from this process include:

- Recognition of my own resistance to this process of revisiting, telling, writing and reading my own stories of pain and suffering; then moving beyond that resistance

- Recognition of avoidance as a coping mechanism in my life; coming to a place where I can accept the reality of my experience

- Recognizing my veiled existence; removing my veil in acceptance and recognition of myself in claiming my identity

- Reframing my experiences as I reflected on both the good and the bad of the experience recalled in the stories; and then able to see more completely what the experience was and allow it to speak to me.

Reinterpreted insights in my experience and reflection include:

- Recognition that the experience of healing involves *listening* to my own story

- Recognizing God's hand at work in and through my experience

- Recognition that grief is a life-long process

- Recognition that healing is a life-long process.

As I have reflected on what it was like to revisit periods of time in my life, it has been draining. It has been hard work and like most hard work, it has been rewarding. The rewards have come in a sense of inner strength, along with assertiveness that is new and feels right. It is who I am. I know myself better than I did before. It is rewarding to know that I don't have to be perfect and I like me, for the most part, just the way I am. The healing on many different levels has been richly rewarding. Rewards have come as I have reconnected with family members of my late husband and developed deeper relationships with my sisters and other family members. Besides my own growth and healing, perhaps the greatest rewards have come with knowing that my stories and my growth are already helping others to reflect on their lives and begin to make changes.

I have looked at some of the most significant relationships in my life. I have looked at those areas of my life needing healing and have shared both my pain and my joy. Healing is not complete, for to claim that would be to say I've arrived and I'm not vain enough to make that claim. Healing is a journey that will continue throughout my life and maybe even beyond. Death may be a doorway to even greater healing.

I am a Christian. God is very real to me. My image of God has never been restricted to mirror my earthly father. And yet, there have been those times in my life when I "put God on the shelf" and felt I could do things on my own. There were other times when I didn't want God to be close, times when I feared God would answer my prayers and that scared me. My image of God has always been one in which God was omnipotent and omnipresent, meaning God was very powerful and that nothing, not my thoughts or my actions were ever hidden from God. In our household there were many secrets kept from those on the outside, but never from God. So, why didn't God protect me when, as a child, I suffered abuse?

Didn't God love me? The "Back to the Bible" radio broadcast told me Jesus loved me, and wasn't Jesus God's only son? My image of God was in direct conflict to what I heard and believed in my heart. I put God on the shelf for a number of years in early adulthood. And yet, even at those times I could take God off the shelf when I needed God. In realizing that no shelf could ever contain or restrain God, who is as close as the air we breathe, I could separate the conflictual images I held of God as both judge and friend and accept, in adulthood, the loving God of my childhood. As I sought God more earnestly in my life I came to realize that God was always with me, even in my darkest moments. God revealed God's self to me in numerous ways, some of which are my miracle experiences described elsewhere in this paper or in my stories as they have unfolded.

Through this healing journey I have come to a place where I can truly believe in a loving compassionate, caring God who will never forsake me. Strength, trust, compassion, forgiveness, empathy, love and acceptance are all part and parcel of the gifts God has endowed me with to fulfill God's purposes in my life. This dissertation process has helped me to see those more clearly as I continue on my own healing journey knowing God is with me.

It is my faith that sustains me and through prayerful discernment God has given me the strength to do the necessary work to make this journey; the courage to explore, to write my stories and then to share them with others. "I can do all things through Christ who strengthens me" (Philippians 4:13).

CHAPTER SIX

THEOLOGICAL REFLECTION

This dissertation is a heuristic, self-search inquiry in which heuristics interpret my life through the interplay of my Christian heritage accessing both scripture and genealogy. I hold a christocentric theology and understand Adam and Eve to be essential ties to my Christian heritage. I bring into the mix the eclectic familial traditions of my parents and grandparents from the Roman Catholic Church, the Anglican Church and the United Church. Theological reflection invites me to enrich my experience through what Killen and DeBeer refer to as "the artful practice of bringing my life into conversation with my Christian heritage" (*The Art of Theological Reflection* 143).

Theology is part of the fabric of my life. My lived theology has numerous components including, but not limited to, story theology, relational theology, experiential theology, transformational theology and a theology of forgiveness. I will reflect, in this chapter, on how my lived theologies unfold within the context of my stories and my healing journey.

I recognize that healing is not something I can accomplish on my own. Faith in God and prayer, or communication with God, were essential elements as I embarked on this incredible journey. Flora Litt in *Healing from the Heart* gives us these words of wisdom which mirror my truth:

> Hurts of the past lodged in our hearts, minds, and bodies often need spiritual work to being healing. One way to the "healing of memories"…involves asking Jesus to walk back with us into the wounded places of our lives, places where we experienced abuse, rejection, or abandonment, places which have bound us in darkness and distress of painful memories. As we open ourselves in prayer, Jesus can and does go back with us to bring healing, for Jesus is not bound by space and time as we are (135).

As I drove to Saskatchewan and Manitoba to revisit, write and reflect, faith sustained me and made it possible for me to face whatever was there to greet me. I am reminded of a familiar quote which says, "Help me to remember Lord that there is nothing that I will face today that you and I, together, cannot handle" (http://www.empoweredaddvantages.citymax.com/page/page/659697.htm). I hold tight to that thought. As I struggle with the challenges that face me I remember the Cross, the crucifixion and the resurrection. I know that what I suffer is nothing compared to what Christ did on the Cross for me. As I struggled to comprehend why I needed to go through all the pain of this healing journey, I pictured Jesus at Gethsemane as "He fell with his face to the ground and prayed, 'My Father, if it is possible, may this cup be taken from me. Yet not as I will, but as you will'" (Mathew 26:39) and I pray as he prayed, "God take this cup from me." I find it difficult to say, "Yet, not my will, but yours God." This healing journey is my cross, my crucifixion and my ultimate hope for resurrection. On the road to Golgotha, Simon, a traveler coming in for the Passover, was forced to help Jesus carry his cross. But Jesus had to go to the cross alone. Many people have willingly walked with me but the cross is mine to carry alone. It has been a difficult journey. There were times when I didn't think I had the strength to carry on. Right to the very last paragraph, resistance attacked me. In the final writing I was overcome with feelings of panic and dread at the thoughts that soon my stories would be available for others to read and I would have no control over who was doing the reading. I did not want to finish. I literally had to force myself to get up, sit at my computer and write. It would have been so easy to pull the covers over my head and go back to sleep and forget all about this painful healing journey. I hear the words of Jesus when as he hung on the cross he "cried out in a loud voice, "Eloi, Eloi, Lama sabachtani? – which means, "My

God, my God, why have you forsaken me?" (Matthew 27:46). I envision Jesus as he hung on

the cross through the poetic words of Jean Vanier,

> the pain,
> the excruciating pain,
> the weight of his body
> hanging by his arms
> nailed to the wood,
> unable to breathe with ease …
> Nailed to the cross
> naked, stripped of everything … (*Jesus, the Gift of Love* 127)

My pain was real. Jesus endured his pain for me and so I wrote not only for my own

healing but to help others find the path to theirs.

In Genesis 37, we see, as we do in many stories throughout scripture, each of the

components of story, relationship, experience, transformation and forgiveness present in the

story of Joseph and his family. Joseph's brothers were jealous of his gifts and his relationship

with his father, Jacob. They mocked him, abused him, mistreated him and sold him into

slavery. As the story unfolds we read of the experience and the family dynamics present

within that milieu. We see favoritism and jealousy played out and ultimately we see

relationships healed when transformation and forgiveness take place. I imagine Joseph hated

his brothers and harboured bitterness for many years, just as I have done. By the time his

family came looking for him he had done a great deal of healing. The reunion required

further healing made possible as Joseph saw his life within God's larger pattern. Joseph

became very powerful and held a place of prominence. Instead of bitterness he showed

compassion to his family. He extended grace and forgiveness in the face of sibling rivalry riddled with envy, jealousy, hatred, cruelty and indignity. Relationships were healed and lives transformed.

While I am encouraged by Joseph's story, I see both the similarities and the contrast within my own story. Unlike Joseph, who believed he had special gifts and abilities through his dreams, I knew I was not special. Jacob favored Joseph and because of that favoritism, Joseph's brothers hated him. In reflecting back, I can see aspects of favoritism in the way my father portrayed my scholastic abilities to all his friends and anyone who would listen. I wonder how that favoritism affected my siblings. At that stage of my life, I did not recognize the favoritism for what it was. Joseph took the circumstances of his life and turned them into opportunities. He exercised forgiveness that was totally unexpected. I choose to follow Joseph's pattern and as I do so, instead of harbouring bitterness I will let go and forgive. I have moved through the circumstances of my life and allowed them to shape my life and be the catalyst for growth. The reflection involved in this research has shown me that what entices me to revisit Joseph's story over and over again is my interpretation of the fairytale ending in which the family came together in forgiveness and acceptance of each other and *they all lived happily ever after.* I would have liked that for my family. In reality I revisited my own story, rewriting it as I saw the reality of both the good and the bad. In coming to a deeper understanding of my own truth I discovered a measure of peace knowing that my story is unique to my experience and it matters, to me, to my sisters, to my children and to God.

Story Theology

If we dwell in His story,
in truth are we His disciples,
and we will know the Truth
and the Truth will free us.

(Terrence W. Tilley, *Story Theology* 213).

Story Theology is foundational to the essence of my being. It is an integral part of

my ministry, my life and this dissertation. Terrence W. Tilley in *Story Theology,* introduces

us to this concept by claiming

> *Story Theology* …allows the Christian to evaluate not only the stories which
> constitute the Christian past, but also the stories which offer possibilities for
> reconstructing one's own life in the present. By attending to life-stories and
> considering standards of truth for stories, the ways to come to know the Truth
> and thus be free (John 8:32) can be seen (xix).

In this context, Story Theology is vital to any attempts to theologically reflect as I

look at my stories in relation to scripture and our history. It bears reiteration here as a

reminder that we are our stories. We are the "living human document" (Boisen qtd. in

Asquith 2) bearing witness to each experience in our lives.

As stories in scripture speak to me, I find myself living, at times, in parallel to my

ancestors though Adam and Eve. Tamar, in 2 Samuel, suffered incestual abuse and rape at

the hands of her brother Amnon. I am reminded that dysfunctional families have existed

since the beginning of time and affluence or lack thereof has little or no bearing. Tamar was

the daughter of a King. I was the daughter of a poor farmer. Both of us suffered abuse. In

Tamar's situation, Absalom, another son of King David, eventually kills his brother Amnon

for raping Tamar. This story speaks to my story at many levels. I have learned that incest

and other abuses were rampant in our household and the dysfunction affected every member of the family. Tamar's story invites deeper reflection on the totality of life within that family

circle. I wonder where her mother was while she was being raped. Absalom, while he hated

his brother for what he had done, in a sick way, condoned the rape by saying to Tamar, "Be

quiet, he is your brother. Don't take this thing to heart" (2 Samuel 13:20b). In my own

experience I was unable to speak to anyone for fear of repercussions. I lived under a code of

silence. Absalom learned of the rape and took his sister to live with him. Absalom carried

bitterness in his heart towards his brother and two years later, he chose to respond to the

mistreatment of his sister by carrying out his own acts of violence and killing his brother.

Violence begets violence. I prayed for and dreamt of the death of my brother and when he

died in an accident I felt responsible. I carried that guilt for many years. I let go of the guilt

and the bitterness, partly as I began to speak of the abuse and then more completely as I

wrote and reflected on the reality. Writing the experience was like reaching in and lifting it

out of my heart and placing it on the page. Then I was able to read the experience and let it

read me in a way that proved to be both freeing and healing. There is healing as I move

beyond the guilt to greater spiritual health.

The claims that "God made man because he loves stories" (18), and "God made man

because he loves to share stories" (*Story Theology* 73), at first glance seemed to me to

trivialize creation and God's purposes for humanity. Yet, as I sat with the *story* and looked

at the deeper meaning in reflection, the words resonated within my spirit and spoke to me of

God's interest in my life. God wants me to know God and God wants to know me. As a

Christian I need to look to scripture to understand my past, my present and my future.

Scripture is both God's story and my story.

A children's bible story book that I gave to my grandchildren last Christmas pictured

Jesus surrounded with little children for story time. I also picture my mother gathering her children around as she played guitar and led us in a sing-a-long of gospel and country songs. In "Honor Thy Father and Thy Mother," I have claimed my parents were not much for story telling. But Mom shared her story in different ways. She shared through her life, as it spoke volumes of the difficulties she endured, and she spoke joy through her music. Memories of her music tell me a great deal about her life and her personhood. Her gospel songs speak of her faith while her country music spoke of her love of life. As I look back, I can see her smile and hear her voice in my memory. Mom was, in many ways, a private person but she discovered other ways to share her story and she lives on in my memory and my heart. She too was a victim and I wonder if, like me, she felt invisible or unimportant as she fulfilled the duties of an obedient wife.

As I go back in time and revisit my stories, I can reframe the experience in light of new insights, understanding, wisdom and goodwill that comes with maturity. Reliving the experience of each of my stories and recording them was akin to being freed from a heavy burden. The healing was in both the story itself and in the ability to rewrite those stories in light of reframing them beyond the vision and understanding of my childhood.

Scripture invites us in—to be a part of all that is humanity. In Psalm 78, Asaph reminds us of the importance of repeating the teachings and stories of God's power and faithfulness to the generations that follow.

> O my people, hear my teaching;
> listen to the words of my mouth.
> I will open my mouth in parables,
> I will utter hidden things, things of old—
> what we have heard and known
> what our fathers have told us.
> We will not hide them from our children;

We will tell the next generation.
The praiseworthy deeds of the Lord,
His power, and the wonders he has done (Psalm 78:1-4).

That scripture passage from Psalm 78 is all about sharing the stories of God, listening

to the teachings of God and making sure they are passed on. God is part of my life, part of

my story and I am part of God's story. Since I cannot teach what I do not know, I am

beckoned forth to know and gain a measure of understanding of how God's story and mine

are one and the same. Terrance Tilley, says that

> a factor contributing to the rise in story theology was the recovery of the
> realization that *human* experience is *inherently* narrative in form...Rather than
> think of our experience as timeless points, events or occurrences...we should
> think of experience as patterned in and through time. What this means, then,
> is that experience 'is itself *an incipient story* (*Story Theology* 23).

Through listening to stories and reflecting on our own story we learn about ourselves

and about others. We pass on the stories from generation to generation in various ways, by

word of mouth, by example, and by the written word. Long before the written word people

told stories. This concept can be applied to our lives today and be enlarged to include the

significance of faithfully telling my story in the spirit of Psalm 78, to my children, to my

family and to future generations as we realize the power there is in sharing our stories and

passing them on.

> Stories are the vehicle that moves metaphor and image into experience...
> stories provide a perspective that touches on the divine... of all the devices
> available to us, stories are the surest way of touching the human spirit (Kurtz
> & Ketchum 17).

As we tell our stories and listen to the stories of others our lives intertwine,

our spirits connect and we become part of each other's story.

Relational Theology

Relational theology, which is foundational to me as a person, as a minister, and as a chaplain is a vital component to humanity. Relational theology is "a term that embraces a variety of expressions of emphasis on interpersonal relationships as central to one's theological outlook" (*Dictionary of Theological Terms* 235). Canadian Association for Pastoral Practice and Education training, essential for professional chaplaincy, is based on relational theology. As a chaplain, I enter into relationship with people of all walks of life on a daily basis. God created us as relational beings. "A relationship" says Tom Marshall, "is a mutual sharing of life between two or more persons" (*Right Relationships* 11). He goes on to say,

> The relationship we have with the Holy Spirit is the most intimate of all relationships... The relationship of the Holy Spirit with our spirit is a relationship of "in-being" or mutual indwelling, we are in him and he is in us. He that is joined to the Lord is one in spirit with him ... intimacy at any level is hard won and not without pain. In fact growth and development at any level involves pain and suffering (23).

Do we make sense of our own pain and suffering knowing that it is present even within our most intimate relationships with God through the Holy Spirit? "Kubler-Ross associated suffering with the development of spirituality. 'Nothing is a faster teacher,' she noted, 'than suffering. The more we suffer, the earlier the spiritual quadrant opens and matures'" (Egnew 5). Strong connections are made between the pain and suffering of relationship and personal growth and development. "Suffering is relieved by removal of the threat ... to the integrity of personhood ... and restatement of the previous sense of personhood. *Healing then becomes a personal experience of the transcendence of suffering"* (Egnew 5).

In order to understand a person, it is necessary to know her story, to know the context of her life. *Your Story Matters* was written to encourage people to value their own story through writing.

> When we speak of the *story* of a person's life, we automatically envision not only the individual, but other people, relationships, family connections. Stories have characters with personalities and stories, all their own which weave in and out of each other, forming a tapestry. Each person's story gains meaning and significance by its *relationship* to others' stories (Paul 17).

Story is a dialogue with life in which the story is created through the experience and through the remembering and the retelling of that story. In the retelling of my own stories, I have encountered the stories of family and friends and numerous others who are part of my story but each one has their own story. My story would not exist without theirs.

Relationships vary and operate on different levels. In some ways my relationship with my human parents was similar to my relationship with my heavenly parent. I never felt close to either my mother or my father and was constantly trying to prove my worth. I lived in fear of my father. I lived in fear of God after my brother's death. I never felt good enough and was constantly trying to prove myself. My perfectionism and drive to excel is reflective of my need to prove myself good enough in God's eyes. I know that God accepts me just as I am but it is a struggle for me to let go of the patterns learned so long ago. This inner search has given me new insight and awareness that can foster even greater healing.

Jesus spoke in scripture of relationships of love when asked which commandment was greatest in the law he replied,

> Love the Lord your God with all your heart and with all your soul and with all your mind. This is the first and greatest commandment. And the second is like it: Love your neighbor as yourself (Matthew 22:37-38).

Not all relationships are based on love but there must first be an element of care for relationship to exist. Indifference or failing to care does not foster relationship.

Carl Rogers says, "I find I am more effective when I can listen acceptantly to myself, and can be myself" (*On Becoming a Person* 17). I cannot be myself without knowing who that self is. So, there is an element in which I am called to know myself. This heuristic research is part of that process. Rogers was no doubt speaking as a therapist in relation to his effectiveness as a psychologist working with clients, however, there is great wisdom in knowing and accepting oneself in forming any relationship.

Part of relational ministry, modeled by Jesus and demanded in chaplaincy, is the ability to listen attentively to the stories of others, not only with my ears but also with my heart. There were fourteen people in our family and my relationship with each member was different. I never felt I knew my mom and in my growing up years we had a rather distant relationship. I never felt Mom cared for me and didn't feel loved. I often felt as though I was just one more mouth to feed and one more body to clothe. My mom's sister, my aunty Jean, on the other hand, took time for me and made me feel special. She cared. Mom ignored me and never appeared to have time for me. Towards the end of my mom's life our relationship deepened as in her hospitalization I was privileged to be both her daughter and her chaplain. We spent quality, interpersonal time, sharing our stories and getting to know each other in a way we never had in earlier years. This experience was very much like that described in Egnew's abstract with these words:

> Sharing suffering creates interpersonal meaning and melds the life stories of patient and physician. Creating interpersonal meaning and melding life stories produce a *connexional* relationship, " a mutual experience of joining that results in a sensation of wholeness...Connexional relationships reduce the alienation of suffering. As the physician becomes a part of Patients' life

> narratives and 'experiences with' them…. patients no longer suffer alone…the
> role of the physician-healer is to establish connexional relationships with his
> or her patients and guide them in reworking of their life narrative to create
> meaning in and transcend their suffering (Egnew 6).

The concept of *connexional* relationship in this context is that of physician and

patient. Stephens, however, notes that "You are missing something unless you come not

merely in a professional role but in a role of one human being meeting another" (6). I use

connexional relationship in a broader sense as it fits for me on numerous levels as I believe it

is more than merely the doctor/patient relationship of Egnew's article. My mother and I, as

patient and hospital staff, as patient and chaplain, and as mother and daughter developed this

connexional relationship on three different levels. As mother and daughter we shared our

suffering, hers being physical and mine emotional, brought our stories together and

developed a *connexional* relationship that "reduced the alienation of suffering" (Egnew 6).

Part of my suffering came from feeling unimportant and emotionally abandoned by my mom.

The scripture passage that relates most to this experience is "When… my mother forsake me,

then the Lord will take me up" (Psalm 27:10 AV). It is in reflection that I recognize the full

impact of this reality. Nobody wanted me. I really was unimportant and insignificant. Years

earlier I had accepted that I was special in God's eyes. As mom and I shared our stories I

came to know that I was special in my mom's eyes as well. Our stories melded together in

that "mutual experience of joining that results in a sensation of wholeness" (6). As I reflect

on that special experience I realize how very much I miss her.

Yet there is still another level of possibility for the connexional relationship. As I

entered into heuristic self-search inquiry I had to enter into relationship with myself. I had to

write, dialogue, reflect and then I had to *listen* to my stories. Cassell is quoted as saying "to be whole again is to be in relationship to yourself, to be in relationship to your body, to the culture and significant others. To be whole as a person is to be whole *amongst others"* (Egnew 4). As I came to know myself more fully, the "I-who-feels" connected with the "I-who feels" of myself and I was able to reconstruct my identity, revise my life story, find meaning and experience healing. This fits with Egnew's compilation of meaning around the world connexional. Each of the four levels I have introduced here is important and can contribute to the well-being of other people just as they have for me.

Relationship requires commitment. It is more than mere acquaintance. It is taking the time to get to know others, to listen to their stories, to know what brings them joy and what makes them sad. It is intentionally interacting with their lives and inviting them into yours. The heuristic self-search inquiry process of writing and reading my own stories and then becoming the listener has been my mechanism for intentionally interacting with myself as I enter into a new and deeper understanding of who I am.

The book of Ruth concentrates on the healthy relationship developed between Naomi and Ruth. This relationship developed out of respect, commitment and need. Elimelech, Naomi's husband died in Moab and then ten years later, both her sons, one of whom was married to Ruth, died. The women formed a bond of friendship and support. Subsequently they entered into relationship with Boaz. While I know this relationship is indicative of the culture of that day and is portrayed in scripture as good and healthy, it angers and frustrates me as I look at what transpired. What kind of a woman would send her daughter-in-law to seduce her late husband's brother? What would make Ruth obey her mother-in-law's request that she go to the floor of the threshing room and make herself available to Boaz? Were these choices made out of a need for survival or simply because women were seen to exist for the pleasures of men? I know times were different, or were they? I have always enjoyed reading the book of Ruth because I see in it women of strength, courage and character. It speaks of loyalty, steadfastness, dedication and commitment. But there is more and stories such as this remind me of the need to stand for equality, for what is right and true. "God created man in his own image, in the image of God he created him; *male and female* he created them" (Genesis 1:27), tells me that we, as all of humanity are created in God's image and I believe that means we are created equal. When I look back to biblical times and then to today we, as women, still have a long way to go to achieve equality. But, there was another relationship evident in the book of Ruth. Naomi had a strong relationship to God. Ruth demonstrated the influence Naomi had on her life when she indicated a willingness to pledge allegiance to the God of Naomi, the God of Israel. Naomi's faith had to have shone through to influence Ruth.

My sister, Laurie, is twelve years my junior. She was the pest who became my best friend. I looked after her as a child. She was a delightful child and she was a nuisance in my life. In many ways I took on the parental role and I am aware that my life influenced her, just as surely as Naomi influenced Ruth. When I was in grade twelve I took her to her first day of school. I was the one who would help with her hair as she got ready for school in the mornings. In home economics I made matching outfits for the two of us. I loved my little sister and when I grew up and married she spent summer holidays with us. As she grew to be a teenager and then an adult our telephone bills were horrendous. The bond between us grew even stronger. We shared our lives and our relationship grew from one in which I was her protector and mentor to one of deep respect and equality and we became more than sisters. We became best friends as I imagine Ruth and Naomi to have been.

God has created us for loving relationship and Jesus came to show us the way to enter into relationship through his example. Relationship was the key to his ministry. He interacted with people of all walks of life. He visited with the woman at the well. He went to the home of the tax collector and ate with him. The fact that he was often surrounded by twelve of his closest friends, his disciples, did not preclude him from entering into relationship with others he encountered through his relatively short time on earth. Jesus always had time for people.

My relationship with my earthly father was based on hostility, disdain and fear. It was not what I would have wished it to be. Regretfully, I know I was not as loving as I wished I had been. A number of years ago, I responded to a challenge set forth by Sydney Shelton, in his work, *In His Steps* to ask the question, "What would Jesus do?" before taking any action. I don't recall when I stopped thinking about that but perhaps if I had continued the practice my behavior towards my dad would have been quite different. I can envision sitting down with him and asking him to tell me what life has been like for him without Mom? What was his childhood like? Were his parenting skills, or lack thereof, learned from the examples of his father? Did he, like me, suffer the effects of an alcoholic father? How could I have helped him to find a measure of happiness in his old age?

As I re-vision his story, I can listen and just let it be his story without holding onto the guilt I have carried believing myself to have fallen short of the mark. I can let go and there is healing.

As I reflect back on the healing journey of this dissertation in new retrospect of relational theology, I wonder where God was, at difficult times when my need for God was the greatest? I didn't always feel God's presence. When my dad and grandpa came home drunk and we felt their wrath, where was God? Where was God's wrath against the injustice? My childhood memories are confused as to where God fit in my life. I wanted, so desperately, to experience that loving God of Back to the Bible. The harsh reality of my life seemed to portray God, if in fact God existed, as someone who either didn't care or condoned the violence and unpredictability of alcoholism that was rampant in our household. And so I hid in the fantasy of storybooks and my imagination.

I didn't feel God's presence when my husband died. I felt abandoned. I look back to scripture, especially in Old Testament times and wonder if people like Tamar, Joseph, Naomi and Ruth felt distanced from God. Did they, like me, wonder where God was in the midst of their pain and suffering? Naomi and Ruth both experienced grief as their husbands, like mine, died. Naomi's grief was compounded as both her sons died. I remember my mom's grief when my brother died and know, from the many people I have journeyed with as a chaplain, that losing a child is perhaps more traumatic than anything else. Tamar was raped by her brother and silenced by her family. The horror of that experience would have remained with Tamar all of her life. The silence would have kept her victimized and, from personal experience, I know the shame she must have felt believing the abuse to have been somehow her fault. Joseph, like me, grew up in an extremely dysfunctional family. There was more than sibling rivalry; there was hatred in that household. His brothers threw him into the cistern. (There was no water in the cistern.) We had a cistern at our house and even without water it would have been a musty, cold, damp place. Joseph was literally imprisoned there until his brothers pulled him out and sold him into slavery. I felt imprisoned on our farm and often felt there was no escape. Joseph must have felt helpless and angry in his predicament. He was truly abandoned. These are only a few of the many examples of victimization at the hands of others. I imagine each of these people must have questioned where God was in the midst of their pain and suffering.

Although I have the assurance from scripture that God has not and will not abandon me, that fact did not preclude my moving away from God. The burning guilt I felt in the surety that my prayer had caused my brother's death was my excuse to move away from the loving God of my childhood in whose presence I felt safe and secure. The relationship shifted to one in which God became someone to avoid and to fear. I didn't deny God—but the relationship changed. It was at this time in my life that I became involved in a youth group at church and traveled with my cousins or other neighbors whenever I could attend. I was searching for that loving God of past experience while at the same time pushing away a God who would answer the stupid prayers of a child wishing someone dead. An element of fear had entered the relationship and my relationship with God took on elements of the relationship I had with my human father. I lived in fear of wrath from both of them. Adam and Eve hid, in the Garden of Eden, when their sin was exposed. I hid from God to avoid having to face the reality of having caused my brother's death.

I lived in the midst of confusion and uncertainty around my perception of God and yet sought to know and to be loved by God. This mirrored my experience of living in the chaos of alcoholism and abuse in our household. I yearned for the attention and approval of my dad and yet dreaded his violent and abusive behaviour. Evidence, in scripture and in my own experience, attests to the strong need for us as human beings to connect with God, our maker, in a very relational way. In our finite humanness it can be beyond comprehension to relate to an omnipotent God who is both omniscient and omnipresent and so God came down to earth in the person of Jesus Christ to help us to relate in a real human sense.

Three times in scripture we find the words of God, "I will never leave you nor forsake you." We read of Moses repeating God's words to the Israelites assuring them of God's presence with them always (Deuteronomy 31:6). We find the same assurance being given to Joshua after the death of Moses (Joshua 1:5). In the New Testament, the writer of Hebrews uses the same words in the context of exhortations. After a call to persevere, we are given an outline of what faith is with a quick walk through the Old Testament, which reminds us of some of the people of faith. We are then urged to,

> Keep on loving each other as brothers (sisters). Do not forget to entertain strangers, for by doing so some people have entertained angels without knowing it. Remember those in prison as if you were their fellow prisoners, and those who are mistreated as if yourselves were suffering...because God has said,
>
> 'Never will I leave you
> Never will I forsake you
> So we can say with confidence,
> The Lord is my helper; I will not be afraid
> What can man do unto me? (Hebrews 13:1-3, 5b-6).

Although the words vary slightly they give a sense of assurance that we can be confident that God will be with us through whatever the journey of life holds.

The possibility of abandonment by God is a strange concept to me at this stage of my life. It is not a possibility that my theology will readily accept and yet I am aware that this reality was not always evident in my life, and I have questioned where God was in the midst of my pain and suffering; in those times when I felt abandoned and forsaken. I felt abandoned when my husband died. I felt abandoned by family, friends and God. "For this reason a man will leave his father and his mother and they will become one flesh" (Genesis 2:24) became very real to me. I felt as though my flesh was literally being ripped apart. The physical pain was real. It was the worst pain I have ever endured. It was beyond description.

My grief was so intense that I could not share it with those reaching out to support me. At that particular time, I did not want to be in relationship with anyone, and that included God. The paradox was that I felt so alone and abandoned. Yet scripture assures us that we are not alone and eventually I came back to knowing that God was with me through it all. In reflection I recognize there were numerous times when I moved away from God and then would draw close again. Finally after attending a week-end retreat I knew I wanted God in my life and began to earnestly seek to know God in a personal way.

We bring into each relationship, with God or with others, our humanity with all our preconceived notions and expectations. If we can let go of preconceptions then we can enter into honest and open relationship with God and with others.

> The Bible insists that real communication is possible, not yet perfect or complete, but real; knowledge of persons is possible, not yet perfect but real and meaningful. That is because communication and personal knowledge both existed before man was created, having been from all eternity within the being of God (Marshall 59).

That real communication is essential to relationship building in which we can be the hands, the feet and the heart of God as we reach out to others and bring God's love, which is in us and operational through us as we enter into relationship.

Experiential Theology

> *Experience is, for me, the highest authority.* The touchstone of validity is my own experience. No other person's ideas, and none of my own ideas, are as authoritative as my experience. It is to experience that I must return again and again, to cover a closer approximation to truth as it is in the process of becoming in me (Rogers 24)

Those words are not mine, they are those of Carl Rogers, but they speak of my reality as they so adequately describe the importance and the power of personal experience. Truth is revealed through the lived experiences of our lives and yet our understanding of truth is reshaped as experiences unfold. Experiential theology allows me to invite the interplay with scripture, theologians, and my own life. Experience supports the belief that we are our stories and that God and others are part of those stories

Experience is a powerful teacher. I have heard this referred to as the 'school of hard knocks,' but it is far more than that. Experiential learning becomes even more powerful when in conversation with scripture it becomes intertwined with our beliefs and the image we hold of God. Scripture is full of reports of radical changes in people's lives as they come face to face with the reality of experiencing Jesus in their everyday lives. In John's Gospel, we read of the Samaritan woman and the conversation Jesus had with her at the well. She was an outcast, but Jesus didn't treat her that way. Her personal encounter with the Lord changed her life and as she shared her experience, others were changed. "They said to the woman, 'We no longer believe just because of what you said; now we have heard for ourselves, and we know that this man really is the Savior of the world" (John 4:42). The conviction of spirit involves more than hearing the word. Somehow, in the mystery that is God, the Word becomes real, all doubt is gone and **we know**. This is the tacit knowledge of heuristic research and self-search inquiry.

My earliest perception of God, filtered through my experience of knowing in the depths of my being that God was real, came at about five years of age. I had gotten into the habit of finding a place of seclusion and tuning in each evening to the "Back to the Bible" radio broadcast on Canadian Broadcast Corporation. I loved that program. It spoke to an unfulfilled need in my soul. I devoured the bible stories. I could almost transport myself into the story and I loved hearing about this Jesus who came to walk with us. He loved the little children. I needed that love. I needed to know there was someone out there who cared for me, Marjorie, with my unruly curls, and my tattered hand-me-down clothes. Was it really possible that Jesus could really love all the little children? If so, then that included me. There were only seven (at that time) in our household and there didn't seem to be enough love to go around. I thirsted to hear, over and over again, those assurances that Jesus loved me. I listened to the sweet music in the song "Jesus loves me." I even sang along, although I knew I couldn't sing, but Jesus loved me and I needed to hear my own voice sing those words. As a young child I felt the love of God and knew in my heart that there was a God out there who loved me. I heard the words that Jesus loved me, *just as I was.* I invited Christ into my heart and it felt so good. The Spirit of God reached through those radio waves to touch the heart of a small child, to touch my heart and I knew Jesus loved me.

However, the faith of my childhood did not remain strong. There was very little nourishment for faith to grow to maturity in our household. Without nourishment there is no growth. As my perception of God changed from that of the loving God of my childhood to a God I feared following the death of my brother, I developed a theology of avoidance and simply moved away from God. Over the years, life got in the road. My faith wavered and I had an "on-again off-again" relationship with God as I moved into adulthood. I rationalized a great deal and things had to make sense to me. Sometimes God didn't make sense and I often felt I was on my own. Eventually things happened to change that and bring me back to a personal relationship with Christ.

Personal relationship with Christ through experience also shaped the beliefs of noted theologian, Martin Luther. His 95 propositions (or thesis) posted on the Castle Church door at Wittenberg, in October 1517, may have been the spark that ignited the reformation, but his

own experience of

> being caught in a thunderstorm while walking towards the village of
> Stotternheim at which time, a bolt of lightening knocked him to the ground,
> and Luther, terrified, called out to Catholicism's patroness of miners: "St.
> Anne, save me! And I'll become a monk. ..." (*Church History in Plain
> Language* 256),

moved him to recognizing the importance of experiential theology. It was Martin's personal

experience that ultimately led him to seek deeper understanding of the scriptures and of God.

"A new and revolutionary picture of God began to develop in Luther's restless soul." The

words in Romans 1:1, "For therein is the righteousness of God revealed from faith to faith; as

it is written, the just shall live by faith" (AV), came alive for Luther as he

> saw the connection between the justice of God and the statement that 'the just
> shall live by faith.' Luther grasped that 'the justice of God is that
> righteousness by which through grace and sheer mercy God justifies us
> through faith.' These words spoke to his soul and Luther considered himself
> 'to be reborn and to have gone through the doors into paradise…the cross
> alone can remove man's sin and save him from the grasp of the devil' (257).

Luther's experience seems to parallel that of Saul in Acts as on the way to Damascus,

"suddenly a light from heaven flashed around him. He fell to the ground and heard a voice

say to him, 'Saul, Saul, why do you persecute me?'" (Acts 9:3-4). It took this personal

experience to bring Paul to a radical change in his theology and his life just as it did with

Luther. Paul, named Saul at birth, was a Pharisee from Tarsus. He was a persecutor of the

Christians and yet through personal experience, as Jesus appeared to him on the road to

Damascus, he was convicted and became a powerful disciple of Jesus.

Another pioneer theologian, whose experience directed his theological path, was John

Wesley who played a huge role in the Methodist revival or awakening in England following

sixteenth-century reformation and seventeenth-century Puritanism. "On May 24th, 1738,
while listening to the reading of Luther's preface to his *Commentary on Romans,* Wesley's
heart was 'strangely warmed,' and he trusted Christ alone for salvation from sin. His brother
Charles had had a similar experience two days earlier" (*Christianity through the Centuries*
393).

      Years ago, as I worked through Bittner's, *You Can Help with Your Healing,* I once
again drew close to God and Christian community. On a Good Friday, in a small chapel in
Gaetz Memorial United Church in Red Deer, the small congregation in attendance shared
communion and I experienced Christ. As I went forward to receive communion, God met
me at the altar and I left that service different than when I came in. It is hard to explain. I
just knew I had encountered Christ through the Holy Spirit once again in my life, and I was
reminded of the scripture in which Jesus tells us "And I will ask the father, and he will give
you another counselor to be with you forever…I will not leave you as orphans (John 14:16 &
19). This time there would be no turning back and never again would I deny God's rightful
place in my life.

      My experiences have been different from those of Martin Luther, the Apostle Paul
and John Wesley but God has revealed God's self to me just as surely as he did to them and
experiential theology is a reality in my life. God meets us where we are at particular times in
our lives. Jesus is real in my life and I know that the experience he suffered in death on the
cross was real. The cross experience was for me. "For God so loved the world (that includes
me) that he gave his one and only Son (to die on the cross) that whoever believes in Him
shall not perish, but have eternal life" (John 3:16).

As chaplain, I have felt the unmistakable presence of the Holy Spirit as I kept vigil with family members of a dying patient. A particular patient's wife and children watched in awed silence as the sun broke through on that cloudy day, rested on the face of their loved one for a brief period and then just as he breathed his last and his spirit departed from his body, the sun disappeared and the sky again became overcast. I am convinced; God is present in our midst.

> Otherwise they might see with their eyes,
> Hear with their ears,
> Understand with their hearts
> And turn and I would heal them (Matthew 13:15b).

Transformational Theology

"...but be transformed by the renewing of your mind, so that you may prove what the will of God is, that which is good and acceptable and perfect" (Romans 12:1-2).

Transformation signifies change. It is indicative of a shift; a difference in our way of being; a change in perception or belief. It is the ongoing natural process throughout our lives, through which life's experiences change us. There are those transformations that we welcome and those which are uninvited and not of our own choosing. While Biblical terminology looks to transformation as change for the better, there are many examples throughout the scriptures that speak of transformation not of the person's choosing. Much of the healing in my journey would not have taken place without recognizing the impact of those uninvited, unwelcome transformations and looking back at how they have shaped my life.

Sexual abuse transformed me from an innocent child to a guilt-ridden, shame-filled girl who believed it was my fault and that somehow I was evil. Tamar, King David's daughter, experienced a similar transformation (2 Samuel 13). Both of us were robbed of our childhood, of our innocence and our rights to safety and protection within the family setting. Those experiences shaped my life and are forever a part of who I am. Faith, strength of character, determination, perfectionism, stubbornness and the ability to escape to my own dream world became survival techniques, which have stood me in good stead throughout much of my life. Even as I grew in maturity and relative wholeness the experiences and their effect on my life remain part of who I am. Ultimately I allowed transformation of a new kind to unfold as I made informed choices in regards to how I would live and interact with the effects of those experiences. If I were to extrapolate from Tamar's experience I would choose to imagine her becoming a strong woman of faith and courage who developed the ability to stand up to the male counterparts in her family. That would have been extremely hard at that time in history, more so even than in my time. But imagination allows us to tell the story and create a desirable ending.

Sharing my stories for the first time was part of the process of my healing transformation, which allowed me to move out from under the veil of secrecy into a place of authenticity and freedom. Ultimately my healing journey involved coming into a renewed, deeper relationship with God, working through *You Can Help with Your Healing*, entering ministry, Clinical Pastoral Education, (CPE) training, Christopher Leadership involvement, and numerous other positive influences over a period of many years.

Being 'transformed by the renewing of my mind' indicates an acceptance of distinct possibilities of momentous changes in attitude. So, what was it that renews my mind to the point of change? It was going back to revisit the old family farm and allowing Matheu's joy to penetrate my heart. It was writing the stories of a painful childhood, allowing the memories to fill in the gaps and then reframing and rewriting the story from a different perspective. DeSalvo reminds us of transformation when she says

> According to Japanese literary theorists, like Zeami Motokeyo, 'writing cleanses the mind, enables the writer to achieve serenity, for it purges us of *tangled emotions.'* The writer then is inevitably changed by the act of writing (70).

As I laughed and played with Matheau, running through the grass and exploring the old farm, my hatred and anger dissipated as I saw through his eyes and remembered not only what I hated about that place, but the very things I loved. I remembered the joyful times and finally could see a different picture than the one I held in my mind for many years. Pent up hatred and anger were released; my soul was purged of the tangled emotions and I was 'transformed by the renewing of my mind' (Romans 12:1-2).

The past five plus years have been a continuous transformative journey. The dissertation process has challenged me to authenticity. It has invited and forced me to look closely at who I am and what forces drive my life. The sense of being driven, developed in my formative years, is alive and well.

As I began the process I had it all neatly mapped out. I completed all the required courses in two years and fully anticipated completing a doctorate in a maximum of three years. I was merely jumping through the hoops to achieve. The process itself was not in my scope of vision. There came a point however, in which I had to accept that my projected deadlines were not going to materialize. In reflection, I am reminded of the concept of Alcoholics Anonymous in which, recovering alcoholics often have to 'hit rock bottom' before they realize that they cannot do it on their own. In a way, I believe I hit my own rock bottom before I came to realize that I needed to shift my "attitude of certitude" (Killan & DeBeer 4) and transform my vision and direction for my dissertation. I came to a place of knowing that I could not continue on the path I had set. It was a hard reality check for me. It was decision-making time. Was I willing to let go and let God?

Through a lengthy process of prayerful discernment, the ability to listen, truly listen to the wisdom of others, slowly enveloped me. I began to hear what I did not previously have ears to hear. The emergence of the knowledge that my dissertation had to be a heuristic research/self-search inquiry, a study of myself, came slowly at first and then began to take shape. As it formed in my mind, it also formed in my heart and I was able to get real with myself. I was revitalized with a new excitement. I was re-energized as I focused on my own life and the healing stories that emerged from my years of experience. The change was significant. The letting go was enormous. I surrendered my all to God and the feasibility of healing became an actuality.

Karl Rahner, an influential Catholic theologian, describes the resurrection of Christ as the greatest transformation in all of Christianity. Harvey D. Egan, S.J, in his biography of Rahner quotes Rahner as saying,

> Christians confess that God's saving power raised the crucified Jesus bodily from the dead…In his whole historical reality Jesus has risen to glorified, transformed perfection and immortality, thus the risen Christ is neither a resuscitated corpse nor a spiritual idea but the fully transformed Jesus (*Mystic of Everyday Life* (136).

In scripture we read of the transforming of our earthly bodies into glorified bodies as we make that journey into eternity with God.

> For our citizenship is in heaven, from which also we eagerly wait for a Savior, the Lord Jesus Christ; who will transform the body of our humble state into conformity with the body of His glory, by the exertion of the power that He has even to subject all things to Himself (Philippians 3:20 -21).

This is the ultimate Christian hope for the future, but we live in the world today where transformations happen to everyday people in everyday lives much as they did in biblical times. We don't always recognize transformation. As I wrote my "Heuristic Reflection" chapter, inadvertently, I wrote "hallowed" when I intended to write "hollowed" in reference to the feelings I experienced inside as I read the words of Orual in Lewis' novel, *Until We Have Faces*. Both words, hollow and hallow are important to my story and my reflection. Stories are hollow and meaningless when they are missing their core or incomplete. As I am open to listen to and articulate my stories they become hallowed (holy) in completion. Stories become holy and whole when they come from openness and vulnerability rather than from the places of secrecy. Perhaps as I remove my veil of secrecy and come out of hiding, my face, too, will be seen by God to be hallowed. I am holy in God's sight.

The Apostle Paul speaks of transformation as he reminds the Christians of Corinth that our lives are to reflect the glory of God as through the Holy Spirit we become more Christ like and thus we live more Godly lives.

> But we all, with unveiled face, beholding as in a mirror the glory of the Lord, are being transformed into the same image from glory to glory, just as from the Lord, the Spirit (2 Corinthians 3:18).

My unveiled face is the removal of the secrecy around my childhood and the invitation to look closely at who I am. It is freedom to be me, to live a Godly life and have God's love reflected through me to all whose lives intertwine with mine. This is my desire.

Forgiveness

"Forgive us our trespasses, as we forgive those who trespass against us" (Matthew

6:12) (KJ). These are powerful words from the Lord's Prayer. I memorized these words

from the King James Bible in grade school and am not sure I ever knew or understood the

concept of what those words really meant. We pray and ask forgiveness of God in relation to

the forgiveness we grant to our *debtors* (terminology from the NIV). The concept makes

perfect sense. The actual doing is more difficult.

Forgiveness is "to cover; to expiate; to lift up; to relieve; to release and to pardon"

(*The New Strong's Complete Dictionary of Bible Words* 103). Forgiveness is a learned,

intentional action in which I must decide, based on my own free will, to forgive someone

who has wronged me. Likewise, I must accept forgiveness extended to me for the wrongs I

have committed. With God's help both of these become distinct possibilities. In the Lord's

Prayer we pray that God will "forgive us our trespasses as we forgive those who trespass

against us" (Matthew 6:12 AV). The shed blood of Christ on the cross covers our sins and

we are forgiven. If I 'lift up' to God in prayer and release the actions of those I need to

forgive, forgiveness removes my need to judge the actions of others and begins the healing

process that brings freedom from carrying burdens of unforgiveness in my heart.

Alastair Cunningham claims, "Forgiving others is almost universally recognized as a

noble human capacity" (*Bringing Spirituality into Your Healing Journey* 89). He explores

true forgiveness as opposed to "pseudo forgiveness," which, in effect, says "I can forgive you

because I am superior to you" (90). Cunningham quotes Paramahansa Yogananda from his

commentary on a major Indian spiritual text, the *Bhaqgavad Gita*, with these words of

wisdom:

> Forgiveness in the man (person) of God consists of not inflicting, or wishing
> to inflict, punishment on those who harm or wrong him/her. She/he knows
> the cosmic law will see to it that all injustices are rectified; it is unnecessary
> and presumptuous to attempt to hasten its workings or to determine their
> form…this is not to say that wrongdoers should have no curtailment (but)
> those whose duty it is to enforce just laws…should mete out (justice) without
> malice or a spirit of revenge (89).

It is our responsibility to forgive without retribution and without wishing harm to the

person we need to forgive. We need to forgive from a position of equality, not superiority.

This is a tall order. As I reflected on the memories and images evoked by reading my stories

I realized that one of the hardest things I ever had to do was forgive a monetary debt owed to

me by one of my brothers. (Perhaps that's an indication of the materialism I lived out of at

the time.) Relationship had become strained between us. I had loaned him a considerable

amount of money, which he appeared to have forgotten. There were many occasions when I

could have used that money and several times I asked him to make payments. He never did

and eventually I was so burdened by the debt that I was uncomfortable in his presence.

Heaviness weighed on me as I sat in judgment on his failure to pay the debt. Family

gatherings were difficult when both of us were there. In his presence the debt overshadowed

all other thoughts as I became obsessed and could think of nothing else. Why didn't he ever

acknowledge the debt? It was truly as though he had forgotten it. This went on for a number

of years until, with a group from my church, I worked through Vernon Bittner's guide, *You*

Can Help with Your Healing, in which the Serenity Prayer is prayed together each night:

> *God grant me the serenity to accept the things I cannot change,*
> *Courage to change the things I can, and*
> *The wisdom to know the difference* (6).

As I prayed this prayer and the words pierced my heart, I realized that I could not

change my brother, nor could I force him to make restitution without taking him to court and

I had no desire to do that. I could only precipitate a change in myself. As this prayer spoke directly to my heart, so did steps eight and nine of the process. Step eight calls me to make a list of all persons I have harmed and become willing to make amends to them. Likewise I was asked to make a list of all those who had harmed me. Step nine then calls us to make amends wherever possible to those we have harmed and confront those who have harmed us. My brother was on the top of my list. I knew instinctively I had to face my brother and confront him. Attempts to discuss this matter with my brother had 'fallen on deaf ears.' I decided to make a trip to Saskatchewan to resolve the matter. As I drove the six hours to our family farm, which was where my brother lived, I heard an audible voice telling me to forgive the debt. At first I was stunned, and then I realized that God was speaking to me. "Forgive the debt," the voice said. Over and over again the voice rang in my head until finally I pulled over on the side of the road and wrote a letter to my brother which I ended by writing, "Paid in Full" in huge letters across the bottom of the page. I explained to my brother that as a Christian I could no longer carry the burden of that debt and needed to forgive it in order to move on in spiritual growth and personal healing. My brother was not home so I delivered the letter and as I drove home that night I felt as though a huge burden that I had carried for far too long had been lifted. The letter was never acknowledged. For me it didn't need to be. At last I was free.

One of the additional benefits from having forgiven my brother was that it freed me to be totally honest in my response to family members when they inquired about the debt, which they did because it was not a secret that he borrowed the money. My response now was, "The Debt's been paid in full."

Over two thousand years ago, as Christ died on the cross, my sins were forgiven and "Paid in Full" was written in the book of life next to my name. "Forgive us our debts as we forgive our debtors" (Matthew 6:12), takes on a deeper meaning as I realize that the debt I forgave pales in comparison to what God, in God's grace and mercy, did and continues to do for me.

Hendrikus Berkhof connects healing with forgiveness as he explores the compassion and the message of radical forgiveness brought to us by Jesus.

> God directs himself with his condescension to a helpless world, estranged from him, which is particularly represented by two groups, by the guilty and the wretched. To the guilty, Jesus comes with the message of radical forgiveness. 'For the Son of man came to seek and to save the lost' (Luke 19:10), and to the wretched he comes with the deed of compassion. 'When he saw the crowds, he had compassion for them, because they were harassed and helpless, like sheep without a shepherd' (Matthew 9:36). This compassion is shown especially in the many healings Jesus performed. Both forgiveness and healing aim to elevate man, on the basis of God's gracious coming, to the true humanity of being a free and happy child of God (*Christian Faith* 301).

Jesus came with that message of radical forgiveness to the woman caught in adultery. Jesus said, "Go now and leave your life of sin" (John 8:1). Not one accuser remained after Jesus had challenged them to cast the first stone if they themselves were without sin. That same message of forgiveness is for me today.

My dad was a person who held grudges all his life. He was never able to forgive and was not able to accept forgiveness. He did not believe God could forgive him for the things he had done in his life. He carried the guilt and would not let go of it. He could not forgive himself. He also never forgot the injustices against him and would repeat them often to us as his family. When his parents died he received nothing while his two sisters inherited the house in British Columbia. My dad had the family farm but, he would remind us, he had

paid for it many times over with the rent he paid to grandpa. To my knowledge, my dad
never let go of the bitterness he harbored and in all probability carried that with him to his
grave. Dad kept a running ledger of all the wrongs committed against him. Even his good
friends did not escape his verbal wrath. (Of course, it was to our listening ears, not theirs.)
He could not find it in his heart to forgive, either himself or others. He never talked about it
but I wonder if he ever forgave Gordon, the thirteen-year-old who was driving the truck in
the accident in which my brother Bill was killed. I will never know.

  As I reflect on forgiveness in my own life, I wonder—how does one forgive the dead?
And further, how does one ask forgiveness from the dead? As I look to forgiving my
brother, I know I can confront him in creative visualization. I want him to say he is sorry. I
want him to tell me why he did those things to me. I am not quite ready to face him in my
imagination and so I lift it up to God in prayer and release his actions and the healing process
that brings freedom in releasing the burden on my heart can begin. The abuse I suffered at the
hands of my brother is not easily forgotten, but forgiveness is something I am called to in the
words of the Lord's Prayer. At times I believe I have forgiven him, but then there are those
times when I know I still hold some of the anger in my heart. I want to be able to confront
him and ask him why he did those terrible things to me. Bittner's work reminds me of the
importance of confronting those who have harmed me. There are ways to do that in absentia.
In facilitating grief groups, I invite participants to write letters to those who have died. It is
the writing that is important. It allows for previously unsaid things to be spoken through the
written word. The healing aspect of story is duplicated in this process. Writing it all out,
asking the why questions, writing the hurt, the anger and the frustrations can help the healing
process to begin. One day I will do that. I am not sure what the letter will say but I am sure I

will ask him why he did the things he did. Why did he hurt me so? There is still work to do in that area. I am not quite ready and for now, I am content with that.

Asking forgiveness is perhaps more difficult than granting forgiveness. As I reflect, I am aware that, even in her death, I need to ask forgiveness from my mom. As I spent time with her in the final stages of her life and we shared the stories of our lives, I felt guilty for my response to her illness over the years and yet I did not mention it. Step eight in Bittner's guide (78) calls me to list those I have harmed and become willing to make amends to them. Mom was sick a lot of the time as I was growing up and I resented having to take responsibility for my siblings. I believed her to be a hypochondriac and I know my actions portrayed my disgust. I was not the least gracious in helping out at home. I now believe that my mom probably suffered from clinical depression and perhaps post-partum depression. My mom is no longer alive but I need to take steps to seek forgiveness anyhow. I so appreciate the precious time Mom and I shared towards the end of her life and now will write to her apologizing for my ungrateful attitude and mean spirit towards her. I wished I had done this while she was alive but it is never to late to seek forgiveness and I can continue my own healing journey.

"Be kind and compassionate to one another, forgiving each other, just as in Christ God forgave you" (Ephesians 4:32).

Summary

Theological reflection is a natural part of the heuristic self-search inquiry research process. "What is the experience of healing as revealed through story?" when put into a theological context brings together the threads of my life. Theology refers to "the study of God and God's relation to the world" (Webster's 1223). Each of the themes explored in this chapter invited me to look at what the scriptures had to say, what theologians had to say and then reflect on how my experience fit with those concepts.

We are our stories and God is part of our story just as we are part of God's story. We are created beings, created by a God who, according to Paul, writes because God wants that story to be recorded for all people for all time (22). We are encouraged by Psalm 78 not only to share God's story but also to teach it to all generations. Stories allow us to understand our lives in relation to our Christian heritage (Killen and DeBeer 143). Our stories matter and our stories gain meaning and significance in relationship to the stories of others (17). Story theology is the encompassing medium that reveals relational theology, experiential theology, transformational theology and a theology of forgiveness as my experiences unfold.

Nouwen speaks of the wounded healer having to bind his own wounds and at the same time be prepared to heal the wounds of others. Jesus' broken body has become the way to health (*The wounded Healer* Nouwen 82). Because I have experienced much of the pain and grief of those I minister to I become the wounded healer and am able to come alongside them in their need. It is essential to first enter into relationship with those you would journey with. Sharing suffering brings lives together in a sensation of wholeness (Egnew 6). As my eldest son and I shared a memory book honouring his dad and then recently journeyed together to Uncle Sternie's funeral we have drawn closer together in a sense of wholeness.

Experiential theology started for me at age five when I first felt the indwelling of the Holy Spirit within my soul and knew God loved me. God has revealed God's self to me in various ways and at various times throughout my life. My relationship with God, not being nourished, did not remain strong and needed healing. At a Good Friday Service I had an experience not unlike that which Luther described in which his heart was "strangely warmed" (*Church History in Plain Language* 256). My heart was deeply touched and my relationship with God began the necessary restoration process.

I am continually being transformed by the renewing of my mind (Romans 12:1-2). This dissertation process has been transformational for me as I have shifted from my attitude of certitude to a more open stance in which I can listen and receive. The very act of writing changes the writer (DeSalvo 70). It is not, however, only the act of writing that effects change but rather it is also the reflection, the reading and the sharing that affect change and can be the catalyst for healing.

Forgiveness has been a stumbling block for me. Working through Bittner's guide is the first memory I have of intentionally working through a process of forgiving someone. It is much more than a simple response to "I'm sorry." It takes work to forgive but with these words we are admonished by scripture to do just that, "And when you stand praying, if you hold anything against anyone, forgive him, so that your Father in heaven may forgive you your sins" (Mark 11:25).

EPILOGUE

Two or three things I know, two or three things I know for sure,

and one of them is that to go on living I have to tell stories,
that stories are the one sure way I know to touch the heart
and change the world" (Allison *Two or Three Things I Know for Sure* 29)

The journey has been incredible. But in the final analysis, what does it all really mean? The words of Dorothy Allison, quoted above, aptly speak to the importance of story and allude to the healing aspect in the broadest sense of changing our world. Her words speak to the power of story.

This final chapter will summarize my discoveries in response to my question, "What is the experience of healing as revealed through story?" In this research process I have looked to what the literature has said on healing in relation to story and weighed that in light of my own research in which I reflected on my experience of healing as revealed through the stories of my life. My stories were those in which I experienced pain and suffering through grief and loss, poverty and abuse, perceived neglect and memories held onto for too long. Throughout my research process these truths were confirmed for me:

Healing Restores Fragmented Relationships

I experienced this to be true. Towards the end of my mom's life a relationship that was almost non-existent was healed as we spent precious time together and shared our stories. We became mother and daughter with a closeness I could not have even dreamt of previously. This is what Maddix and Soles referred to with their words, "Healing brings the fragments of our life together as a whole (Maddix & Soles 11).

Healing Constructs the New from the Old

As my sisters and I have shared our stories of living with the affects of alcoholism and abuse we have developed new relationships based on mutual understanding , trust and love. We have become more than sisters. We are friends who share many things. What began as one weekend together and a sharing of memories has grown into a yearly sisters' weekend as the five of us "getaway" just for fun. Wolin and Wolin describe this experience as, "Healing is building a new world from the ruins of the old (177).

Telling the Story Changes our Perception

I visited the family farm with my grandson, Matheau and that experience became one of my stories for this research. Through reflection and writing, my perception of the farm changed drastically. I was able to frame my memories differently to see both the good and the bad. I no longer dreaded the farm and more pleasant memories became part of my reality. Stone claims that the very act of telling the story not only changes our perception but it changes us (47). In my experience I changed as a result of a combination of things. Firstly I revisited the farm, and then I reflected on that visit, wrote about it, reflected some more and slowly my perception changed as I saw through the eyes of my grandson and allowed the new experience to permeate my being. There was a change in me and I could go look forward to going to the farm.

The Wounded Healer

I am the wounded healer. As hospital chaplain I journey with people in times of
sickness, pain, grief and death. I believe God works through my experiences to make me a
better chaplain. My pain and woundedness can become "a major source of healing power"
(*The Wounded Healer 83*).

The wisdom of Henry Nouwen says, "Do not run, but be quiet and silent. Listen
attentively to your own struggle. The answer to your question is hidden in your own heart
(*Reaching Out* 35). Moustakas says "concentrated gazing" (39) is one of the crucial
processes of heuristic research and the focus of the investigation should be "the inverted
perspective" (15) which really means we look in ourselves to discover our answers. The "I-
who-feels"(Sela-Smith 85) has searched deep in my heart, in those secret places, to bring
forth the answers to my question and to allow those answers to bring me to a state of
wholeness.

Learnings and Contributions

This chapter will also speak to the contributions made to the greater community and
how my ministry is enhanced as a result of my self-search inquiry.

The "things I know for sure" (Allison 29) that have been re-enforced through this
work, are that my stories are important. I know that there is freedom in being able to put
voice to our stories. There is opportunity to reframe our experience in light of the theological
framework of God's grace, which allows us to see the broader picture and know that we, as
human beings, are ultimately connected and that life in all its complexity reflects God and
God's work.

> I see myself as a witness with a public purpose. I write about, what I have
> lived through—experiences that might not be commonly known—to heal
> myself. But I also write to help heal a culture that, if it is to become moral,

ethical, and spiritual, must recognize what these writers have observed, experienced, and witnessed. I write to right a human wrong—one that affected me surely, but one that affects others, too (DeSalvo 216).

I know that this research experience has changed me. I am different. I can repeat with confidence the words of Carl Rogers, "I am enough" (http://www.irishhealth.com/index.html?level=4&id-5002 3). I view life differently than I did five years ago as I began this journey. I am more compassionate. I have found my voice and am able to reveal my face to the world.

> In his final novel, 'Till We Have Faces,' Lewis powerfully presents the following proposition: In order to see the face of the Divine, we ourselves must have a face. The search for God and for our own identity is, in the end, intimately interwoven (Praying with C. S. Lewis 102).

I write to bring new life to a smothered spirit, to hidden memories that weigh as dead weights until the new reality is reborn through writing. The old self is re-membered and becomes the new self revitalized through knowing and accepting that there is much more to my story as I alter my perception and see through different eyes, through the eyes of my understanding, the eyes of my soul. It is then that I can grow and move towards that wholeness described by Maddix and Soles (10).

In getting to know and understand myself at a deeper level, I am able to see God through different eyes, through the eyes of my soul. I see God reflected in my father's eyes, in his searching, in his loneliness and in his pain. I am able to put my memories in perspective and recognize that while indeed some of them were painful, ultimately they are all part of who I am and in that I can declare, "I count it all joy" (James: 1-2), in which joy is not seen as the absence of suffering but rather the presence of the Lord in my life. I can see God's handiwork as that which I have endured is used to encourage others to look at their own experience and grow to wholeness through telling, through writing and through sharing

those experiences. DeSalvo in *Writing as a Way of Healing*, speaks of the healing benefits of

sharing our work while still cautioning us to,

> care for ourselves as we make our work public…Vicious criticism reinforces
> the writer's deep-seated fear that the story shouldn't be told, that the story
> isn't important, that the story won't be believed. Vicious criticism can silence
> stories that must be told (210).

As I found my voice, I also found the courage to share and reveal much that had been

hidden for so long. I started out as a victim. I became a survivor in the sense of "continuing

to survive" (DeSalvo 215) in which I employed whatever strategies necessary to cope with

life on a daily basis. As I overcame obstacles I became a conqueror and finally, as more than

a conqueror in Christ Jesus, I claim to be a witness. This is my transformative journey.

> Being a witness to our experiences, though, means taking on the responsibility
> of telling what happened to us—writing a historical record, a public
> document. The "witness," …offers testimony to a truth that is generally
> unrecognized or suppressed (DeSalvo 215).

This dissertation is my public document, my testimony to my experiences. In the

Pentecostal Assemblies it is common to give testimony to the transformations in our lives

through the working of the Holy Spirit. We do this publicly in front of the entire

congregation. My congregation is all those who will read my dissertation. Ric LaPlante's

desire for me was that I would become a better Pentecostal. This is the fulfillment of that

desire.

This dissertation specifically set out to explore the experience of healing as revealed

through story. Although the heuristic research/self-search inquiry was a look at my personal

experience, the readings I have done indicate that many peoples' experiences resonate with

my own and attest to the fact that we are indeed our stories. People such as Loiuse DeSalvo,

Matthew Fox, and Susan Paul, among others, recognize and have written on the deep connection between healing and story and the importance of sharing our stories.

DeSalvo speaks directly to some of what I feel as I complete this work knowing it will be published. There is a queasy feeling in the pit of my stomach as I think of people reading some elements of my story that I would just as soon not have written. I am painfully aware of the possibility of sharing parts of the sacredness of the stories of others as my story overlaps with theirs. And yet I plunge on knowing that I must as I hold onto the words, "The truth shall set you free" (John 8:32), and trust that in reading my story, my truth may also set others free to explore and tell their stories. If my healing and stories contribute in some small way to one other person's healing, then the goal of this dissertation will have been met.

A quote from Henry Miller in a letter published in *Art and Outrage,* spoke of how much writing had changed him.

> The more I wrote," he said, "the more I became a human being. The writing may have seemed monstrous (to some), for it was a violation, but I became a more human individual because of it. I was getting the poison out of my system (*Writing as a Way of Healing* 4).

Miller's words explain the healing component present in writing the healing journey. Telling the story is the antibiotic required to release that infection that becomes poison from pent up, hidden, hurtful, memories that infect every aspect of our being until at last the burden is lifted and we are free to be whole.

Matthew Fox says, "The healing process of making whole and integrating also includes a return to one's origins" (*Original Blessing* 121). I have done that by going back to those times in my life of greatest pain and challenge. I have reflected on where I have come from, where I am now and what the future holds.

Inner healing, for me, is heart surgery with the biblical image of a heart of stone being replaced by a heart of flesh (Ezekiel 11:19). My heart was softened as I revisited places that held painful memories for me. As I reflected and wrote my stories, then read them, firstly to my sisters, and then aloud to myself, my stories were the conduit for healing. This was the crescendo, the climax of my experience.

My heart has been softened in renewal and change. Healing continues to allow me to move forward and let go of what was. Healing invites me to a change in attitude and a shift in perspective as I try to understand my parents, my siblings and even God. Healing for me is moving 'out of the box.' It is taking feelings stored inside and releasing them. It is acceptance of what is past. It is stepping out with renewed hope and anticipation of the future. It is a sense of well-being. There is a peace in knowing that all is well with my soul.

I am no longer the person I used to be. I have changed. I have discovered the secret of letting go. That letting go involves searching my memories to identify the lies I have fed myself and lived under over the years. As I look squarely at the reality of what was and allow it to surface without fear, then I can look to forgiving, knowing that I am forgiven by God through Christ on the Cross, and forgetting the past as I press on to the high calling of Jesus. It is a choice I make to no longer hold onto the old identity of who I believed myself to be with all the lies of *no-good Whitfield brat, never amount to anything, failure,* as I choose to put on a new reality and allow myself to be truly transformed by the renewing of my mind. In the letting go I have been transformed in ways that allow for things to unfold, to experience my own story anew and let it speak to my life. In many ways I have died to the old self I used to be. I have been through the fire and yet have not been consumed, have been scorched, but not burned beyond recognition. As I lived through the indignities of poverty, alcohol abuse, death of a brother, death of a husband and journeyed through each experience I exited the other side, ready to take on the next experience. Healing did not happen overnight and was not always recognized at first glance, but as the stories are retold and I look back at the experience, I see that I am changed and I journey forward with renewed strength. I can see clearly now, in retrospect, that "… in all things God works for the good of those who love him, who have been called according to his purpose" (Romans 8:28).

In my own healing journey, I have learned to be in the struggle and wind my way through it – emerging on the other side a stronger, healthier individual. As the writer of Hebrews declares,

> therefore, since we are surrounded by such a great cloud of witnesses, let us throw off everything that hinders and the sin that so easily entangles, and let us run with perseverance the race marked out for us. Let us fix our eyes on Jesus, the author and the perfecter of our faith … (12:1-2a).

My research question was "What is the experience of healing as revealed through story?" I have learned to live in the question. It is through sharing our stories that we connect and that healing opportunities unfold. It is through revisiting our stories that it is possible to change our perception and see through new eyes of understanding. It seems somehow fitting that as this work draws to a close and I have revisited those most painful times in my life, including grieving the loss of a husband, that I now, too, grieve the loss of my brother-in-law Sternie. Sternie died December 26th, 2005 as this dissertation drew to a close. It was a difficult task to officiate at his funeral and yet it was good. It was good to revisit the stories and allow healing to begin anew. It was good to be reminded that those whose lives intersect with our own are forever a part of us.

Since this was a very personal journey and a look at my own healing, there was a need to look at what the process was for me. In order to heal, there must be something to be healed from. Some of my journey reflected healing already in process while some healing continues today. Writing itself was a freedom. It was a way of letting go of secrets held inside for too long.

Rachel Naomi Remen, M.D. says, "Curing is the work of experts, but strengthening the life in one another is the work of human beings... Sometimes the deepest healing comes from the natural fit between two wounded people's lives. It makes one wonder about the source of such healing" (*My Grandfather's Blessings* 213). God created us to be in relationship, in community with one another. It makes sense that such strengthening and healing would be part of the greater plan for our lives as we interact and enter into relationship and become part of the stories and the lives of others.

Exhilaration arises within me as I look ahead to what contribution can be made to the larger community. I recognize that my struggles are analogous to those of many others. Personal breakthroughs can assist others in finding their way to healing and wholeness. As Allison so eloquently put it, "Stories touch hearts and can change the world" (86). It is the hope and belief of this writer that my stories will "read the reader" which is a concept explored by Steiner as he speaks of the story engaging and challenging the reader (18). Perhaps they will provide a *natural fit* between my life and the life of another wounded human being. If so, they may remind others of their own stories, give them the encouragement to explore those stories and connect with the healing aspects and the significance of knowing that each individual's story matters. Story gives voice to that which is otherwise unheard or unspoken. Story can bring freedom and allow the teller to release hidden wounds and feelings.

The world doesn't change overnight, but if I can somehow modify my little corner of the world, and everyone else does likewise, we can make the world a better place in which to live. Father James Keller, a Maryknoll priest and founder of the Christopher movement and subsequently the Christopher Leadership Course often said, "It is better to light one Candle than to curse the darkness" (*To Light a Candle, the Autobiography of Fr. James Keller* 114). Father Keller adopted this saying from an old Chinese Proverb and eventually it became the motto for Christophers'. Christopher means Christ Bearer and we can all be that by sharing our stories and helping to heal the world. The Christopher Leadership course played a significant role in my life. It has encouraged me, both as a student and now as an instructor, to develop my own self-confidence through the help of others and then reach out to help make my corner of the world a better place in which to live. As an instructor I am privileged to journey with others as they discover their own self-confidence by recognizing that each of us is special. We have God given gifts and abilities and potential to become the best *me* I can possibly be.

In writing the experiences I encountered ethical dilemmas that pushed me to explore beyond the boundaries, to expand my own horizons and then look beyond the approaches of either Moustakas or Sela-Smith. I solicited the assistance of an ethicist as I inserted an addition step into my methodology, which gave me the confidence I sought to enable me to reveal family secrets in a sensitive and compassionate manner. I relied heavily on the *Health Ethics Guide* and utilized the methodology developed and reprinted with permission in chapter three of this dissertation.

As Paul states, "Each person's story gains meaning and significance by its *relationship* to others' stories" (17). My stories would have no meaning if not intertwined with the stories of family, friends and neighbors whose lives have intersected with mine. I am no longer the person I was as a young girl living on that Saskatchewan prairie farm. Life's experiences have shaped my life. They helped me to become the person I am today, being stronger, more compassionate, more understanding of others and better able to cope with whatever life holds in store for me because of the building blocks created through the many relationships that have helped in the creation of my life story. I no longer live in that place of hurt and sorrow that I claimed as a child, a teenager and a young adult. Today I am a happy, mature adult, content in the knowledge that healing is ongoing. I am blessed beyond imagination and know that if I were to die tomorrow, I do so, having lived a full, rich live. I know I will experience further pain and suffering. It is part of the reality of our human condition. By the grace of God, if I am open to the experience I can be open to the ultimate journey towards wholeness.

I have a new sense of inner peace. I am more accepting of life with all its curves. I am able, although it is still difficult and at times forced, to flow with the process.

I am able to perceive myself reaching the goals I set for myself without fear of failure. I have heard that success is failure turned upside-down. What has precipitated that change in me? Prayerful discernment would be number one. Through research and reflection I have come to know and understand who I am and am able to accept my gifts and limitations. I like myself and believe that with God's help I can fulfill the plans God has for my life. The support of family and friends has given me the strength and encouragement I have needed to travel this difficult healing journey.

I can declare with confidence that this dissertation is exactly what it needed to be at this particular juncture in my life. All the changes, in committee and in direction have been beneficial. The process has forced me to be introspective and has allowed for a depth of understanding of myself that will be beneficial in my life and my ministry. I have changed in the process. I have changed in how I see things. I am able to reflect theologically at a deeper level and to see the face of God in others and the hand of God in life and all of creation. My worldview is bigger than it was before. I am more understanding and more compassionate of those whose perception differs from my own. I am a work in progress and can "run with perseverance the race marked out for us" (Hebrews 12:1b). The race is not yet finished. I am a better chaplain, a better minister, and a better person. I am a better chaplain in knowing the power of story. I am a better minister as I listen more intentionally with both my ears and my heart. I am a better person in knowing that my stories are not mine alone but can serve to encourage others to reflect on their experience, to not remain stuck in the past, but to utilize their stories to move forward into wholeness and health with confidence and hope. I operate, as a person, more completely out of the all of who I am. I recognized this change in myself recently when as guest speaker at a Christopher banquet at the Bowden penitentiary, I shared with inmates that they too could change their perception of their life's story by revisiting it and seeing through different eyes just as I had in my chapter "Through the Eyes of a Child." I was able to share with them the importance of our stories and how we can utilize them for personal change, healing and growth. Afterwards a number of the graduates approached me to thank me and let me know that my story spoke directly into their lives. It encouraged them and brought a sense of hope. They could relate. Moments such as these give me the assurance that the purpose of this dissertation is already beginning fulfilled.

My journey to wholeness is reaching far beyond personal growth and satisfaction as the

benefits reach others in my sphere of influence.

> When we defeat the still, small voice of God inside us, we lose. But that
> voice inside us will not be stilled forever…it will find a time when we are
> vulnerable. It will attack us at a weak moment. And when the struggle is
> over, we will like Jacob/Israel be *bruised* and limping. But again like Jacob,
> we will be whole, we will be at peace with ourselves, in a way we never were
> before (Harold S. Kushner, *Living a Life that Matters* 127).

WORKS CITED

Allison, Dorothy. Two or Three Things I Know for Sure. New York: Dutton, 1995.

Anderson, Herbert and Edward Foley. Mighty Stories, Dangerous Rituals. San Francisco: Jossey-Bass, 2001

Asquith, Glen H. Editor. Vision From a Little Known Country: A Boisen Reader. Decatur: Journal of Pastoral Care Publications, Inc., 1992.

Bartlett, John. Familiar Quotations, A Collection of Passages, Phrases and Proverbs Traced to Their Sources in Ancient and Modern Literature. 16th ed. Boston: Little, Brown & Co., 1992.

Berkhof, Hendrikus. Christian Faith, An Introduction to The Study of The Faith. 1979. Grand Rapids: Wm. B. Eerdmans Publishing Co., 1990.

Berry, Wendell. Remembering. San Francisco: North Point Press, 1988.

Bittner, Vernon J. You Can Help With Your Healing. Minneapolis: Augsburg Press, 1993.

Bromley, Geoffrey W. Editor-in-Chief. Bible Encyclopedia. Vol. P. 1915 Ed. Howard-Severence Company. Grand Rapids: Wm. B. Eerdmans Publishing Co., 1988.

Buechner, Frederick. The Sacred Journey: New York: Harper San Francisco, 1991.

Cairns, Earle E. Christianity Through The Centuries. Grand Rapids: Zondervan Publishing House, 1954. Grand Rapids: Zondervan Publishing House, 1981.

Catholic Health Association of Canada. Health Ethics Guide. Ottawa: Publication Service of The Catholic Health Association of Canada, 2000.

Cunningham, Alastair J. Bringing Spirituality into Your Healing Journey. Toronto: Key Porter Books, 2002.

DeSalvo, Louise. Writing As A Way Of Healing. Massachusetts: Beacon Press, 1999.

Egan, Harvey D. Karl Rahner, Mystic of Everyday Life. New York: The Crossroad Publishing Co., 1998.

Epp, Theodore, Back to the Bible. CKOM, Saskatoon. 1948.

Fox, Matthew. Original Blessing. Santa Fe: Bear & Co., Inc., 1983.

Fox, Michael J., perf. Back to the Future. Dir. Robert Zemeckis. Universal Studios, 1989.

Graham, Rochelle, Flora Litt and Wayne Irwin. <u>Healing from the Heart</u>
Kellowna: Wood Lake Books, 1998.

Gula, Richard. <u>Reason Informed by Faith.</u> New York: Paulist Press, 1989.

Keller, James Fr. <u>To Light a Candle, The Autobiography of Fr. James Keller.</u> Garden City:
Doubleday & Company, Inc., 1963.

Kennedy, Eugene. <u>If You Really Knew Me, Would You Like Me?</u> Valencia: Tabor
Publishing, 1975.

Killen, Patricia O'Connell and John DeBeer. <u>The Art of Theological Reflection.</u>
New York: Crossroads Publishing, 2000

Kirkwood, Neville A. <u>Pastoral Care in Hospitals.</u> Harrisburg: Moorehouse
Publishing, 1998.

Kubler-Ross, Elizabeth. <u>On Death and Dying.</u> New York: Macmillan Publishing Co.,
1969.

Kurtz, Ernest and Katherine Ketchum. <u>The Spirituality of Imperfection.</u> New York:
Bantam Dell Publishing Group, 1992.

Leman, Dr. Kevin. <u>The Birth Order Book.</u> 1985. Grand Rapids: Fleming H. Revell, A
Division of Baker Publishing Group. 2005.

Lewis, C. S. <u>Till We Have Faces, A Myth Retold.</u> Orlando: Harcourt, Inc., 1956.

Maddix, Thomas D., and Ian C. Soles. <u>Journey to Wholeness.</u> Ottawa: Novalis, 2003.

Maley, Michael, PhD. <u>Living in the Question.</u> Minneapolis: Bodysmart Publications, 1995.

Martin, Charlie. "Young Christian's Forum." <u>Prairie Messenger.</u> 15 June. 2005: 1st Section.

Metzger, Deena. <u>Writing for Your Life.</u> London: Harper Collins Publishers, 1992.

Midler, Bette. "The Rose." By Amanda McBroom. <u>The Rose.</u> 1983.

Mish, Frederick C, editor. <u>Webster's 9th New Collegiate Dictionary.</u> Springfield: Merriam
Webster Inc., 1987.

Morrison, James Dalton, editor. <u>Minister's Service Book.</u> New York: Harper & Brothers
Publishers, 1937.

Moustakas, Clark. Heuristic Research, Methodology, and Applications. Newbury Park: Sage Publications, Inc., 1990.

Moustakas, Clark E. The Touch of Loneliness. Englewood Cliffs: Prentice-Hall, Inc., 1975.

Moyers, Bill. Healing and the Mind. New York: Bantam Doubleday Dell Publishing Group, 1993.

McKim, Donald K. Westminster Dictionary of Theological Terms. Louisville: Westminster John Knox Press, 1996.

Nouwen, Henry J. M. The Wounded Healer. New York: Doubleday, 1972.

Paul, Susan. Your Story Matters. Richland: Inner Edge Publishing, 1997.

Pettinger, Marj. A Family Affair (Jorie's Story). Edmonton: Jorie Publications, 2002.

Powell, John. SJ. The Christian Vision. Boston: Argus Communications, 1984

Powell, John. SJ. Why am I Afraid to Tell You Who I am? Grand Rapids: Zondervan Publishing House, 1999

Remen, Rachel Naomi, M.D. My Grandfather's Blessings. New York: The Berkley Publishing Group, 2000

Rogers, Carl. On Becoming A Person. Boston: Houghton Mifflin, 1961

Rondo, Therese A. Grief, Dying, and Death. Champaign: Research Press Company, 1984.

Sela-Smith, Sandy. "Heuristic Research: A Review and Critique of Moustakas' Method." Journal of Humanistic Psychology 42.3 (2002) 53-88.

Sheldon, Charles. In His Steps. 1896. Ed. Westwood: Barber & Co., 1990.

Steiner, George. Errata. London: Phoenix, 1998.

Stone, Richard. The Healing Art of Storytelling. New York: Hyperion, 1996

Strong, James, LL.D., S.T.D. The New Strong's Complete Dictionary of Bible Words. Nashville: Thomas Nelson Publishers, 1996.

Taliaferro, Charles C. Praying With C. S. Lewis. Winona: St. Mary's Press Christian Brothers Publications, 1998.

The Holy Bible- New International Version. Grand Rapids: Zondervan Publishing House, 1984.

The Holy Bible - King James Version. Nashville: Thomas Nelson Publishers, 1972

Tilley, Terrance W. Story Theology. Wilmington: Michael Glazier, Inc., 1985.

Vanier, Jean. Becoming Human. Toronto: House of Anansi Press Limited, 1998.

-------- Jesus the Gift of Love. London: Hodder and Stoughton Ltd., 1988.

Whitfield, Charles L. M.D. Healing The Child Within. Deerfield Beach: Health Communications, Inc., 1989.

Wilkinson, John. The Bible and Healing A medical and Theological Commentary. Michigan: Wm B. Eerdmans Publishing Co., 1998.

Wolin, Stephen and Sybil Wolin. The Resilient Self: How Survivors of Troubled Families Rise Above Adversity. New York: Villard Books, 1993.

Empowered ADDvantages LLC. 2003. Portals of Prayer. Inspirational Quotes. 12 Oct. 2005 <http://www.empowerdaddvantages.citymax.com/page/page/659697.htm.>

Irish Health. Ed. Fergal Bowers. 25 June 2003. Special Olympics, Croke park, Dublin. 18 Sept. 2005. <http://www.irishhealth.com/index.html?level=4&id=5002>

Journey in Word. Ed. Coyote McRaven. 2002-2005. 15 Nov. 2005 <http://www.spiritsong.com/quotes/>

OTHER WORKS CONSULTED

Au, Wilkie. By Way of The Heart. New York: Paulist Press, 1989.

-------- The Enduring Heart. New York: Paulist Press, 2000.

Buechner, Frederick. Telling Secrets: New York: Harper San Francisco. 1991.

Casarjian, Robin. Houses of Healing: A Prisoner's Guide to Inner Power and Freedom. Boston: The Lionheart Foundation, 1995

Chittister, Joan D. Scarred By Struggle: Transformed by Hope. Ottawa: Novalis, St. Paul University, 2003.

Dossey, Larry. M.D. Healing Words. New York: Harper San Francisco, 1993.

-------- Prayer is Good Medicine. New York: Harper San Francisco, 1996.

Eisner, Elliott. The Enlightened Eye. New Jersey: Prentice-Hall, Inc., 1998.

Fox, John. Poetic Medicine, The Healing Art of Poem-Making. New York Penguin/Putman Inc., 1997.

Framo, James L. Ph.D. Family-of-Origin Therapy, an Intergenerational approach. New York: Brunner/Mazel Publishers, 1992.

Goldenberg, Irene and Herbert. Family Therapy, An overview. Los Angeles: Brooks/Cole, 2000.

Hart, Larry D. Truth Aflame. Nashville: Thomas Nelson Publishing, 1999.

Jones, Paul W. Theological Worlds. Nashville: Abingdon Press, 1989.

Kuhl, David. M.D. What Dying People Want. Canada: Anchor House, 2002.

Lee, Bernard J. and Michael A. Cowan. Dangerous Memories. Kansas City: Sheed & Ward, 1986.

Lemon, Dr. Kevin. The Real You, Grand Rapids: Fleming H. Revell, A Division of Baker Book House Co., 2002.

Lewis, C. S. A Grief Observed. 3rd ed. London: Latimer Trend & Co. Ltd., 1961.

-------- Surprised By Joy. London: Harper Collins Publishers, 1998.

Luepnitz, Deborah Anna. The Family Interpreted. United States Library of Congress: Basic Books.

Moustakas, Clark. Loneliness. Detroit: Prentice-Hall, Inc., 1961.

-------- Loneliness and Love. Englewood Cliffs: Prentice Hall, Inc., 1972.

-------- Phenomenological Research Methods. Thousand Oaks: Sage Publications, 1994

Muller, Wayne. Legacy of the Heart. New York: Simon & Schuster, 1992.

Napier, Augustus Y. and Carl A. Whitaker. The Family Crucible. New York: Harper & Row Publishers, 1978.

Oden, Thomas C. Pastoral Theology, Essentials of Ministry. San Francisco: Harper Press, 1983.

Padovano, Anthony P. Free to Be Faithful. Paramus: Paulist Press, 1972.

Panteleo, Jack P. "The Opened Tomb." The Other Side. Vol. 28, No.2 (March-April 1992):8

Remen, Rachel Naomi, M.D. Kitchen Table Wisdom. New York: Riverhead Books, 1996.

Rich, Phil. EdD, MSW and Stuart A. Copans, MD. The Healing Journey, Your Journal of Self-Discovery. New York: John Wiley & Sons, Inc., 1998.

Roach, Simone M. C.S.M. Caring from the Heart. New Jersey: Paulist Press, 1997.

Samuels, Michael. M.D. and Mary Rockwood Lane, R.N., M.S.N. Creative Healing. New York: Harper San Francisco, 1998.

Satir, Virginia. Peoplemaking. Palo Alto: Science and Behaviour Books, Inc., 1972.

Sela-Smith, Sandy. "A Demonstration of heuristic self-search inquiry: Clarification of the Moustakas' Method." Diss. Saybrook Graduate School, 2001.

Smith, Christine M. Risking the Terror: Resurrection in This Life. Cleveland: Pilgrim Press, 2001

Swift, Catherine. C. S. Lewis. Minneapolis: Bethany House Publishers, 1989.

Swinton, John. Resurrecting the Person: Friendship and the Care of People with Mental Health Problems. Nashville: Abingdon Press, 2000.

Unger, Merrill F. Unger's Bible Dictionary. (Third Edition) Chicago: Moody press, 1966

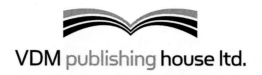

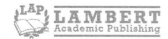
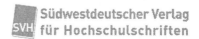